The Hidden Cause of
ACNE

"This intriguing personal account of one woman's experience with acne is a detailed case report that could have been published in the peer-reviewed literature. Using scientific deduction, careful observations, and self-experimentation—a process used by Nobel Laureates such as Barry Marshall, Werner Forssmann, and Ralph Steinman—Melissa Gallico figured out that the cause of her chronic acne was the fluoride added to her drinking water. The fact that other people who read her book also report that their acne cleared up when they switched to fluoride-free beverages and foods suggests this is an area that deserves rigorous clinical investigation."

HARDY LIMEBACK, D.D.S., PH.D.,
HEAD OF PREVENTIVE DENTISTRY AT THE
UNIVERSITY OF TORONTO (RET.) AND PAST PRESIDENT
OF THE CANADIAN ASSOCIATION FOR DENTAL RESEARCH

"This is an astounding piece of work and a 'must-read' for people wanting the true story about how and why and to what terrible effect the addition of fluoride to drinking water is having. As Gallico's riveting personal story attests, public water fluoridation is, in essence, a hazardous waste management tool that is damaging our health in ways we have yet to fully comprehend. Her deep research into this area and the clear, arresting manner in which she presents it is a valuable, even crucial, contribution to ending the antiquated and dangerous practice of adding fluoride to public drinking water."

BILL HIRZY, PH.D.,
SENIOR SCIENTIST AT THE EPA (RET.)
AND PAST PRESIDENT OF THE
EPA UNION OF PROFESSIONAL EMPLOYEES

"Melissa Gallico has authored an engaging book, one that is enjoyable to read despite the seriousness of the subject matter. As she notes, 'it doesn't take a degree in medicine' (or dentistry or science) to appreciate the importance of personal observations in matters of personal health, or to understand the potential consequences of one-size-fits-all medication of the public through the drinking water supply. Fluoride sensitivity (including dermatological, endocrinological, gastrointestinal, and other effects) has been in the medical literature for decades, unrefuted, and deserves the wider awareness that Gallico's work will bring."

KATHLEEN M. THIESSEN, PH.D.,
SENIOR SCIENTIST AT OAK RIDGE CENTER FOR RISK ANALYSIS
AND COAUTHOR OF THE NATIONAL RESEARCH COUNCIL'S
2006 REPORT FLUORIDE IN DRINKING WATER

The Hidden Cause of
ACNE

How Toxic Water
Is Affecting Your Health and
What You Can Do about It

MELISSA GALLICO

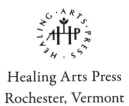

Healing Arts Press
Rochester, Vermont

Healing Arts Press
One Park Street
Rochester, Vermont 05767
www.HealingArtsPress.com

SUSTAINABLE FORESTRY INITIATIVE

Certified Sourcing
www.sfiprogram.org
SFI-00854

Text stock is SFI certified

Healing Arts Press is a division of Inner Traditions International

Note to the reader: *This book is intended as an informational guide. The remedies, approaches, and techniques described herein are meant to supplement, and not to be a substitute for, professional medical care or treatment. They should not be used to treat a serious ailment without prior consultation with a qualified health care professional.*

Library of Congress Cataloging-in-Publication Data
Names: Gallico, Melissa, author.
Title: The hidden cause of acne : how toxic water is affecting your health
    and what you can do about it / Melissa Gallico.
Other titles: End of acne
Description: [Second edition] | Rochester, Vermont : Healing Arts Press, [2018] | Revised
    edition of: The end of acne : how water is the cause of the modern acne epidemic, and the
    cure / Melissa Gardner. ProjectFree, LLC, 2016. | Includes bibliographical references and index.
Identifiers: LCCN 2017042624 (print) | LCCN 2017045471 (e-book) |
    ISBN 9781620557099 (paperback) | ISBN 9781620557105 (e-book)
Subjects: LCSH: Acne—Alternative treatment. | Water—Toxicology. | Fluorides—
    Toxicology—Health aspects. | Fluorides—Toxicology—Nutritional aspects. |
    Skin—Care and hygiene. | BISAC: HEALTH & FITNESS / Healing. | HEALTH &
    FITNESS / Alternative Therapies. | MEDICAL / Alternative Medicine.
Classification: LCC RL131 .G35 2018 (print) | LCC RL131 (e-book) |
    DDC 616.5/3—dc23
LC record available at https://lccn.loc.gov/2017042624

Printed and bound in the United States by Lake Book Manufacturing, Inc.
The text stock is SFI certified. The Sustainable Forestry Initiative® program promotes sustainable forest management.

10 9 8 7 6 5 4 3 2 1

Text design by Virginia Scott Bowman and layout by Debbie Glogover
This book was typeset in Garamond Premier Pro with Gotham, Kepler Std, ITC Legacy
Sans Std, and Briem Script Std used as display typefaces

To send correspondence to the author of this book, mail a first-class letter to the author
c/o Inner Traditions • Bear & Company, One Park Street, Rochester, VT 05767, and we
will forward the communication, or contact the author directly at
Melissa@ProjectFree.Me.

To my mother

*. . . behind all your stories is always your mother's story,
because hers is where yours begin.*

MITCH ALBOM

Contents

Foreword by Stephen Harrod Buhner   ix

INTRODUCTION
Once Upon a Time   1

PART ONE

Cause (*n.*)

1. Why Kitavan Islanders Don't Have Acne,
   but Americans Do   10

2. F: The Invisible Element behind the
   Modern Acne Epidemic   32

3. Rethinking the Cause of Your Acne   52

PART TWO

Affect (*v.*)

4. Stopping Breakouts Before They Start   86

5. Healing Breakouts Overnight   143

6. Becoming Acne-Proof   172

AFTERWORD
The End of Acne   222

∽∽∽∽

APPENDIX
The Plan   229

Acknowledgments   230

References   233

Index   254

*Don't forget about this part —it's important!

Foreword

A NUMBER OF YEARS AGO I wrote a book on the crafting of nonfiction. It was a labor of love (never destined to sell as well as my work on Lyme disease or the treatment of resistant bacteria). Still, it remains to this day my personal favorite. So, it is especially gratifying that every so often someone writes me to say they've been inspired to write their own book. And every so often, someone follows up by asking to send me a copy of the book they have written. Nevertheless, when I received Melissa Gallico's email, and finally reached its lower reaches, its working title was less than imposing: The End of Acne.

My book on the crafting of nonfiction (*Ensouling Language,* Inner Traditions, 2010) plays in some depth with the subtleties and beauty of language, examining in detail the steps involved in evoking its luminous possibilities. So, it was with some trepidation that I said, "Sure, send me the book." When it arrived, and I finally found some time to spend with it, the trepidation had, if anything, increased. "How," I wondered, "could anyone write a fascinating account of acne . . . or its end?" Determined to make my best effort, I grimly prepared myself for a short but tiresome slog through dense, unpoetic prose.

Some two hours later, when I finally awakened from the pages in my hands, I found I had been on a rather incredible journey. The writing was truly enjoyable, the topic engaging, and the implications rather far-reaching. Still, the most riveting element of the book was the mind of the author, whose clear thinking shone through the text in a way that

I rarely experience, even in writers much more seasoned than her, some of whom are quite famous.

Gallico takes you on a journey into the murky world of some rather common medical unclarities. Many medical interventions, formulated in the late nineteenth and early twentieth centuries, were based on quite erroneous premises. The understandings of the day could not have foreseen the pervasive physiological impacts of minute traces of chemicals in our waters or that many substances that were, at the time, thought to be benign are anything but. Nor did they foresee the tremendous ecological impacts (both micro and macro) that corporate capitalism would have on our world in their drive for profits from the production and distribution of chemicals, including those we know as pharmaceuticals.

Gallico's clarity of thought, her penetrating perceptions about the impacts of some of these chemicals on our lives (honed in her work as an intelligence specialist for the FBI), illustrates just how problematic some of the medical science that shapes our lives is. And, as well, the tremendous damage it can sometimes do to the people who live in the midst of the stories it tells. Stories that, as is inevitable with these kinds of things, are altered by new understandings all too slowly.

From the first paragraphs the power of her storytelling is manifest. "Our understanding of the world is shaped through story," she begins. And from there the story she found in her search to understand what had been happening to her unfolds. It's compelling. You hold in your hands the earliest work of a writer that the world needs to hear more from. I hope you enjoy her company as much as I did. Her voice resonated in my mind for months afterward. I hope, too, that if you suffer from the kind of damaging acne that she struggled with for much of her life, you, too, will find surcease in the solutions she offers. You have an able guide in Melissa Gallico.

STEPHEN HARROD BUHNER,
AWARD-WINNING AUTHOR OF 19 BOOKS, INCLUDING
HEALING LYME, THE SECRET TEACHINGS OF PLANTS,
AND *PLANT INTELLIGENCE AND THE IMAGINAL REALM*

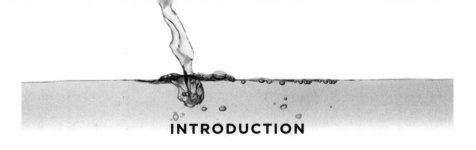

Once Upon a Time

WE TELL OURSELVES science is king, but our understanding of the world is shaped through story. We tell stories about the past and call it history. We tell stories about the present and call it news. Our stories about how to act, think, and live are called culture. And our stories about how the natural world works are called science.

We can tell science is a story because of how it changes over time. The Earth is flat. Now it is round. Airplanes are impossible.* Now they are commonplace. The natural world didn't change, but our understanding of it did. It would be naive to think our current story is a complete picture of how things are.

Every story has a storyteller. Like a musician conjuring a new piece of music into existence, it is the storyteller who decides who the main characters will be, where the story will start, how it will end, and every detail in between. The storyteller is responsible for deciding which storylines to pursue, which to disregard, and which will be overlooked entirely. In most cases, a story has multiple storytellers whose voices weave together in a cacophony of overlapping assertions and ideas. It is up to the audience to decide which version to retell.

---

*Lord Kelvin, an esteemed mathematical physicist regarded for his work formulating the first and second laws of thermodynamics, declared in 1895, "Heavier than air flying machines are impossible." Eight years later, the *Wright Flyer* took flight.

THE STORY OF ACNE

The story of acne commonly told today goes something like this: when your pores become clogged with dead skin cells and other debris, they trap oil and bacteria in your skin causing an infection in the form of a breakout. The story has variations. Sometimes hormones are involved, sometimes they are not. Sometimes genetics are involved, sometimes they are not. Sometimes diet is a trigger, but everyone is different. One aspect shared by these acne stories is the lack of a happy ending—there is no cure for chronic acne, only ongoing treatment.

With the story of acne, the dominant storytellers are dermatologists. As physicians who specialize in disorders of the skin, dermatologists pull their main characters from the pages of their textbooks: pores, skin cells, sebum (oil). The farther away a character is from the skin, the less likely a dermatologist is to include it in the story. Their heroes are chosen from the typical doctor's bag: creams, pills, needles. The antagonists are the villains *du jour:* dirt and bacteria. Dermatologists draw on statistics from the stage as they set it. According to the American Academy of Dermatology's "Acne Stats and Facts" webpage, "85 percent of people between the ages of 12 and 24 experience acne." Is that 85 percent of young people everywhere, or 85 percent of certain young people from a certain time and place?

Another major voice in the acne story is the commercial skincare industry. Together with dermatologists, they are busy researching products and treatments to cure acne and capture a portion of the $120 billion global skincare market. But for a treatment to be profitable, it must be capable of being bottled and sold or administered in a doctor's office. The standards are even higher for the biggest source of funding in acne research: the pharmaceutical industry. If it can't be patented, what's the point?

But what if the cure for acne cannot be bottled, sold, administered, or patented? Would we ever find it? If the main characters are not present on the surface of the skin or even listed on an ingredient label, would we ever notice them?

THE (PARTIAL) STORY OF ME

I am not a dermatologist, an aesthetician, a nutritionist, or any other type of health professional. I'm an intelligence specialist at the Federal Bureau of Investigation (FBI) in Washington, D.C.* You might think I am an unlikely author for a book on acne, but looking back at my career and educational experiences, I now realize they were perfectly tailored to solve a case like this one.

As an undergraduate student at Georgetown University, I majored in Science, Technology, and International Affairs. I am intrigued by the ways we choose to develop our scientific understanding, why certain ideas take hold and others do not, and how the repercussions of scientific advancements are felt on a global scale. I pursued a career in intelligence because, as a young college student in the late 1990s, I looked around at the world and saw terrorism as the biggest upcoming threat to our well-being. After graduation, I entered the United States Navy and later transitioned to the Federal Bureau of Investigation as an intelligence analyst.

During my time at the FBI, I was selected to be a Fulbright scholar at the University of St. Andrews in the United Kingdom, where I worked as a research assistant to Alex Schmid, former head of the Terrorism Prevention Branch of the United Nations. At St. Andrews, I specialized in a branch of International Studies called Constructivism, which involves uncovering hidden assumptions and exploring alternative scenarios through the deconstruction of discourse and linguistics— in other words, the analysis of stories.

After completing my graduate degree in Scotland, I was offered a position at the Boeing Company in Washington, D.C. Most people think of Boeing as an airplane manufacturer, but it also has an Intelligence and Analytics branch. At Boeing, I was contracted to work full time at the FBI, where I instruct an intelligence class at Quantico and travel throughout the country providing analytical support for FBI cases.

---

*The opinions expressed in this book are mine and not those of the FBI.

My area of expertise is helping investigators uncover critical information by assisting them in asking questions. Intelligence analysis involves more than just collecting "the facts" and assembling them into a finished product. People tend to think of analysis as a puzzle, but it is more like trying to assemble a puzzle when half the pieces are missing. Additionally, for reasons that may or may not be malicious in nature, someone mixed in pieces designed to look like they belong to your puzzle when they actually do not. Plus there is no picture on top of the box to guide your efforts.

Whether analyzing the cause of acne or the extent of a terrorist threat, the challenges of thoughtful analysis are substantial. One of the main reasons intelligence analysis is so difficult is because it deals with ambiguous and incomplete data. When we are confronted with inadequate information, we rely on certain subconscious mental processes to interpret it. We want to believe our thinking is guided by rationality and logic, but studies of psychology (and history) show otherwise. The human brain relies not on fact but on mental models—a type of story we tell ourselves—to make sense of the world. These models are essential in the functioning of our daily lives, but they also lead to common cognitive pitfalls. Professional analysts spend their careers trying to develop skill sets to help avoid these analytic traps. We never fully succeed, but gains can be made in trying.

In *Psychology of Intelligence Analysis,* a foundational work in the field, CIA veteran Richards Heuer (2013) explains one of the most fundamental principles of perception that affects analysis: "We tend to perceive what we expect to perceive." (Notice he says we see what we *expect* to see, not what we *want* to see.) This basic tenet of analytic theory is well known, and still we are surprised when we catch it in action, especially in ourselves.

Perhaps the most famous such experiment was conducted by Christopher Chabris and Daniel Simons (2009). If you are unfamiliar with their work, you might find it worthwhile to participate in the experiment yourself by viewing their ninety-second video at www.HiddenCauseofAcne.com/basketball. (But do it now without reading a single word further or else your results will be skewed. Go ahead, I'll wait . . .)

The experiment shows that half of the thousands of people tasked to count the number of passes in a basketball video fail to notice a person in a gorilla suit walking across the middle of the stage and beating his fists on his chest. People who miss seeing the gorilla insist it was not there when they are told about it afterward. As psychologist Daniel Kahneman explains, the gorilla study illustrates two important points about our minds: "we can be blind to the obvious, and we are also blind to our blindness" (2011, 24).

In writing *The Hidden Cause of Acne,* my hope is to make apparent the invisible gorilla on the stage. Once you know to look for him, he is difficult to miss. After struggling with cystic acne for over twenty years, sometimes I wonder myself why it took me so long to put the pieces together. But hindsight is its own type of bias.

Some people might dismiss my experience with acne as anecdotal or balk at the idea of a health book written by a nonmedical professional. My response to such notions is best illustrated with a story.

ENGINEERS AND ANECDOTES: A LOVE STORY

Samuel P. Langley should have invented the airplane. He held an assistantship at the Harvard College Observatory, taught mathematics at the United States Naval Academy, was a frequent guest at the White House, and was named Secretary of the Smithsonian Institution in 1887. In an effort to create the world's first manned flying machine, Langley spent a decade studying the fledgling field of aeronautics research before receiving a grant of $50,000 from the War Department to develop his Aerodrome design. It was the largest research project ever funded by the department at the time. Langley had access to the top scientists in the world and the latest technical research. He had hefty financial backing and the full support of the United States government (does this story sound familiar?). Yet after seventeen years of effort, Langley was unable to figure out one little detail: how to make the darn thing fly.

Orville and Wilbur Wright, on the other hand, had no such competitive advantages. Neither brother had a college education. Technically, they didn't even have high school diplomas. They funded their interest in flying machines with proceeds from their bicycle shop while they worked to build the world's first airplane as a hobby in their spare time. When they wanted information on the latest aeronautics research, their best option was to send a written request to the government via the U.S. Postal Service and hope for a helpful response. Unlike Langley, they weren't even able to bounce ideas off their best friend, Alexander Graham Bell, when they ran into a particularly vexing design challenge.

Yet on December 17, 1903, with the media and all esteemed aeronautical experts noticeably lacking in attendance, the Wright brothers' manned flying machine flew for fifty-nine seconds over the dunes at Kitty Hawk. It took the Wright brothers just four years to create the *Wright Flyer,* but it took the U.S. government nearly forty years to admit the *Wright Flyer,* and not Langley's Aerodrome, was the first manned, powered aircraft capable of flight.

In his bestselling book *Mastery,* Robert Greene explains why the Wright brothers succeeded while Samuel Langley and the U.S. government failed. Langley's team was composed of specialists focused on making the most efficient parts: the most powerful engine; the lightest frame; the most aerodynamic wings. They had an expert military pilot too. This kind of specialization meant the person who designed the wings was different than the person who tested them in the air. Each crew member knew their specialty, but they could only think about how all the parts fit together in abstract terms. In contrast, the Wright brothers personally designed their machine, built it, flew it, crashed it, picked up the pieces, and designed it again. This process allowed them to rapidly uncover flaws in their design and ways to work them out. As Greene states, "it gave them a *feel* for the product that could never be had in the abstract" (2012, 219).

Hopefully the analogy I am drawing between the discovery of the airplane and the cure for acne is starting to become clear. In our story about the birth of aviation (and yes, there are other versions of the story where other flying machines flew first), we see how the Wright brothers' approach was successful because it merged aeronautical theory with the physical world in a way Langley's approach did not. This same approach can be applied to the problem of acne. Greene concludes, "Whatever you are creating or designing, you must test and use it yourself. Separating out the work will make you lose touch with its functionality" (2012, 219). The Wright brothers understood their flying machine from the inside out. It wasn't just something they designed and built. It was something they *experienced*.

The experience of acne is wholly lacking in acne research. Individual accounts are dismissed as anecdotal (in a pejorative sense) and not worthy of consideration in serious study of the subject. Instead of mining anecdotal evidence for clues, acne researchers are preoccupied with producing expensive double-blind, placebo-controlled, randomized trials of prescribable treatments for publication in peer-reviewed journals. Or they focus on statistical analysis of epidemiological surveys that confuse correlation with causation and overlook nuanced complexities inherent in the study of the human body.

Engineers tend not to focus on this distinction between anecdotal and "science-based" evidence. When something seems to work in the real world—even if it was merely "once" upon a time—curiosity takes over and they tinker, test, and repeat until before they know it, they brought a new idea into being. No one told the Wright brothers their flying machine was anecdotal.

As someone who experiences acne, and not just studies it in the abstract, you have an advantage over the entire skincare industry in finding a cure. You can test your theories, make adjustments, and test them again at a pace the "experts" are incapable of matching. You know your test subject better than any outside researcher ever could; its history, its sensations, its environment are all intimately familiar to you.

And because acne is something you experience, you will *feel* when you are onto something or when something is not right even before you identify the reason. In the story of acne, we are not the scientists. We are the engineers.

> *Truth is what stands the test of experience.*
>
> ALBERT EINSTEIN

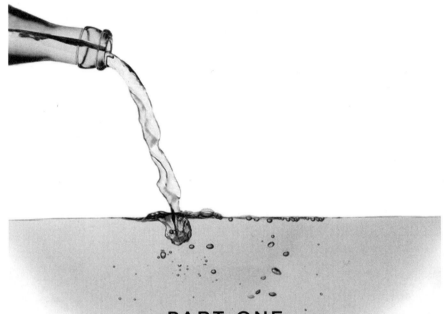

PART ONE

〜〜〜

Cause (*n.*)

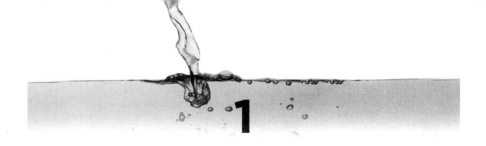

1

Why Kitavan Islanders Don't Have Acne, but Americans Do

BY THE TIME THE SOCIETY for Investigative Dermatology held its sixty-fifth annual meeting in April 2004, they were certain they had the connection between diet and acne long figured out: there was none.

The persistent myth amongst laymen that acne is caused by what you eat was dispelled by science over thirty years prior. Its foundation began to crumble in 1969 when some clever Ivy League dermatologists named James Fulton, Gerd Plewig, and Albert Kigman decided to give sixty-five subjects one candy bar per day for four weeks.* Half the subjects received candy bars with chocolate, but the candy bars provided to the other half of the subjects did not contain any chocolate at all. After four weeks, the researchers did not notice any difference in the amount of acne developed by subjects in the two groups. It was damning evidence for the acne-diet proposition.

---

*To further explore the references cited in this book, please visit www.HiddenCauseof Acne.com/resources for links to journal articles, video evidence, and other resource material. I tried to link to the full text articles when possible, but sometimes only abstracts were publicly available. Oftentimes alumni associations or local libraries will enable you to access full text articles online. Check with your alma mater or your local librarian for more information. The references are also listed in the back of the book.

Just a few years later, a study of twenty-seven medical students provided all the affirmation dermatologists would need to abandon the unprofitable idea that acne is caused by diet (Anderson 1971). The students were asked to identify the single food that was the most likely cause of their acne. It was a multiple-choice question and the possible answers were: (1) chocolate candy bars, (2) peanuts, (3) milk, or (4) Coca-Cola. Each student was then given their suspected culprit food every day for one week. The dermatologist who conducted the study carefully counted and measured the acne lesions on each student before the study began and subsequently on each day of the study as students consumed their particular trigger food. At week's end again the results were clear. Diet does not cause acne.

For the next thirty-four years, not a single acne study was published examining the role of diet. In 2002, Harold Lehman and a team of researchers from Johns Hopkins University conducted a comprehensive review of the scientific literature published on acne during the second half of the twentieth century. The findings revealed 99.6 percent of all acne studies failed to even mention diet, let alone study it as a potential cause of the disorder that affects millions of people each year. This was the prevailing sentiment in April 2004 when the aforementioned Society for Investigative Dermatology invited a nondermatologist, Dr. Loren Cordain, to speak at their sixty-fifth annual meeting.

Despite the title of doctor preceding his name, Cordain was likely the only one in the auditorium that evening without a degree in medicine. He was an exercise physiologist at Colorado State University with a specialty in evolutionary anthropology.

SOMEWHERE OVER THE RAINBOW

Loren Cordain was inspired to apply his knowledge of evolutionary nutrition to the study of acne after reading an obscure article written by Otto Schaefer, a frontier physician who treated the Inuit people in the Arctic for thirty years in the mid-twentieth century. The article, entitled "When the Eskimo Comes to Town," describes the decline in health that occurred when the Inuit people abandoned their traditional diet for modern foods. Acne used to be unknown among Eskimos, but by the time Schaefer published his article in 1971, the change was readily apparent on the faces of Eskimo teenagers. Schaefer states, "One wonders what these people and the other old Northerners would think if they were to read some recent medical publications in which dermatologists belittle or deny the role of dietary factors in the pathogenesis of acne vulgaris."

Intrigued by Schaefer's account of the Eskimo, Cordain searched the scientific literature for more information on how acne is affected by diet and quickly noticed the dearth of research on the topic. He set out to study contemporary nonindustrialized societies who, like the early Inuit, do not experience acne. His inquiry led to Kitava, one of the four major islands in the remote Trobriand Islands of Papua New Guinea in the southwest Pacific. Approximately 2,250 native Kitavans lived on the island at the time, all without access to telephones, cars, or electricity. They subsisted primarily on a diet of fish, tubers, fruit, and coconut.

For his study on acne, Cordain teamed with Staffan Lindeberg, a Swedish medical doctor and professor at the University of Lund who had been studying Kitavan Islanders since 1989. Lindeberg found that the native people of Kitava did not experience diabetes, hypertension, heart disease, obesity, strokes, or acne. During a 7-week period in 1990, Lindeberg visited all 494 houses in Kitava and examined 1,200 Kitavans aged 10 and older for skin disorders on their faces and necks, and for males, on their backs and chests as well. He did not find a single sign of acne in the entire population, including 300 teenagers and young adults between the ages of 15 and 25.

Cordain also teamed with Magdalena Hurtado, who observed a similar account with the Ache hunter-gatherers of eastern Paraguay. The traditional diet of the Ache consisted mainly of wild and foraged foods and select cultivated crops such as manioc, maize, peanuts, and rice. As with the Kitavans, chronic diseases including diabetes, asthma, hypertension, and other cardiovascular diseases were rare among the Ache people. To determine if they also did not exhibit acne, Hurtado and her colleagues observed 115 Ache people over an 843-day period. Not a single case of acne was observed by any of the seven examining physicians throughout the length of the study.

Cordain, Lindeberg, and Hurtado published the results of their research in the 2002 *Archives of Dermatology* with the bold title, "Acne Vulgaris: A Disease of Western Civilization." This was the topic of Cordain's presentation at the Society of Investigative Dermatology's annual meeting two years later. For over an hour, he explained the details of his theory, which held promise for clarifying the recent unexplained rise in adult acne, particularly among women.

In light of the new evidence from Kitava and Paraguay, Cordain reinterpreted the results of the famous 1969 chocolate-bar study as two of the study's authors listened from the audience. *Of course* the study showed no difference in acne between the people who ate the candy bars that contained chocolate and the ones that did not, Cordain explained. Acne is not caused by chocolate. It is caused by *sugar*. Both types of candy bars contained sugar in equal amounts, so they caused acne in equal amounts.

After ruling out genetic factors, Cordain and his team concluded that the reason people in Kitavan and Ache societies do not experience acne is because of their low-glycemic diets. As the theory goes, when people eat high-glycemic foods (e.g., soft drinks, bread, sweets, pasta) their blood insulin levels spike and cause a series of hormonal events that increase the production of testosterone and other growth factors. This hormonal cascade stimulates the excess production of oil and an overgrowth of cells lining the pores, leading to inflammation and the bacterial infections that cause acne.

After Cordain completed his groundbreaking presentation, one of the authors of the chocolate study reached over and shook his hand. "Thank you for correcting our mistake," he said (Oaklander 2014).

In 2006, Cordain authored a book called *The Dietary Cure*

for Acne that outlines his anti-acne diet for the average reader and includes an entire chapter of unsolicited success stories. He also published numerous non-acne books on the nutritional principles he uncovered in his research, referring to his recommended eating plan as the Paleo Diet. Cordain went on to be known as the father of the paleo movement, one of the most popular health movements of the early twenty-first century.

Cordain and his colleagues believed they identified the "holy grail" of acne research. Dermatologists long understood the proximate causes of acne—blocked pores, excess oil, bacteria, and inflammation—but the ultimate cause of acne was admittedly elusive. In 2007, researchers from RMIT University in Australia published studies Cordain would later refer to as "the trump card"—randomized, controlled human trials that prove his theory on diet and acne is correct. When study participants consumed a low-glycemic diet, they exhibited a measurable decrease in acne lesions (Smith et al. 2007a and 2007b). The proof was in the sugar-free pudding.

Cordain's insulin theory showed the root cause of acne is high-glycemic foods. There was just one gorilla-ish problem. In the human trials his associates conducted, acne lesions were observably lessened, but they did not disappear altogether. Likewise, the chapter of testimonials in Cordain's acne book is brimming with phrases like "significantly reduced" and "a big improvement." One person even writes "my acne ALMOST cleared up" two times in his testimonial when he tried to implement the paleo diet on two separate occasions.

Dermatologist Susan Bershad responded to Cordain's article in the *Archives of Dermatology* with an article of her own entitled, "The Unwelcome Return of the Acne Diet" (2003). She points out that some American teens who are not inclined to eat sweets or drink soft drinks consume a relatively low glycemic load yet are still prone to acne.

Was this another instance of a dermatologist's subconscious effort to preserve the future of her profession by sabotaging scientific evidence that diet causes acne? Perhaps, but she had a point.

GORILLAS IN THE MIST

When Cordain, Lindeberg, and Hurtado published their revolutionary paper in 2002 asserting acne is a disease of Western civilization, I was somewhere in the Atlantic Ocean oblivious of the scientific literature on acne and yet busy conducting experiments of my own on a sample size of one. But to know the full story, we need to rewind to a few years earlier.

From my adolescence in suburban America to my collegiate and postcollegiate years in Scotland, the edge of the Sahara, and even months at sea, each of these places offered clues that would later prove instrumental in solving the acne mystery. If you read the story carefully, you will see the gorilla enter stage left and exit stage right no less than *four* times. He even beats his fists on his chest once or twice. See if you can spot him.

Looking back over my experience with acne, it would be difficult to remember when I had it and when I didn't if not for a few bookmarks along the way. I'm sure you know what I mean. The miracle treatment that worked for a while and then somehow stopped working. The unexpected side effects. The flare-ups so sudden and overwhelming you thought your face caught fire. The offhand comments that pierce thick skin then lodge in your memory.

During my adolescent years in the suburbs of Philadelphia, I didn't focus on my acne much. I would not even remember having acne in middle school if not for a particular conversation that stuck in my mind. I was walking back from lunch with a group of classmates when one of them said, "Can you believe Kelly never had a pimple?" The answer was no. I *couldn't* believe it. I remember looking at her in amazement and thinking, how is that possible? Clearly I must have had my fair share of acne already. I just assumed it was a part of life. (Cue the gorilla.)

After high school, I moved to Washington, D.C., to attend college at Georgetown. By the end of sophomore year, my skin was so bad that it was time to see a professional. My consultation with the dermatologist was a blur. I remember him bursting into the exam room, studying my face for a minute (maybe), and then saying a few words to my mother before speaking predominantly to his tape recorder. Even in such clinical terms, it sounded strange to hear someone talk about the placement and severity of my acne as if I was not in the room. Before leaving, the dermatologist handed my mother a prescription for Accutane and a topical treatment along with some cursory instructions. That was the last appointment I ever had with a dermatologist about my acne.

I started taking Accutane the summer before my junior year, which I spent abroad in Senegal, West Africa. After arriving in Senegal, I grew increasingly concerned about the warning label on the bottle about avoiding sun exposure. How do I avoid the sun while living on the edge of the Sahara? My skin had already cleared up, so I took it upon myself to discontinue the medication soon after my arrival. I remained effortlessly free of acne for the rest of the year. I remember thinking, "Wow, Accutane works great!" But that was not the whole story.

After my junior year in Senegal, I traveled to Hawaii to spend a month on the USS *Carl Vinson* as part of my training as a navy midshipman. Even though I had only been back in the United States for a few weeks before leaving for Hawaii, my skin had already returned to full-blown acne mode. After reporting aboard, I visited the ship library to pick up some books to entertain me during my free time at sea. When I returned the books at the end of the month, the library custodian remarked, "Your skin really cleared up since the first time you came in." How do you respond to a statement like that. Thanks? But the jerk librarian was right. Why was it so easy to be acne-free on the ship?

Returning to Georgetown for senior year, my acne returned too. This time I decided to try Proactiv, a skincare system comprised of a daily cleanser, toner, moisturizer, and spot treatment along with a weekly mask to remove the impurities that remained. The active ingredients—mainly benzoyl peroxide, sulfur, and salicylic acid—helped keep my acne under control, but they were no match for what my face would face next.

When I moved to Rhode Island to start my navy career, within days my skin was the worst it had ever been. I had deep cystic welts on my chin, cheeks, forehead, even behind my ears and down my neck. I tried the Murad line. Then Dermalogica. Nothing provided relief. My face burned even when I rinsed it with plain tap water. I started to wonder if something in the water was aggravating my skin. I lived in a historic house in Newport; maybe the pipes were made of lead? I began using bottled water to wash my face and I thought it helped a little, but thankfully my time in Newport was short-lived.

After just six months in Rhode Island, I transferred to Norfolk, Virginia, to report for my first assignment on the USS *Wasp*. I was hoping my skin would clear up on the *Wasp* like it did on the *Carl Vinson,* but no such luck. One day the ship's doc knocked on my door. "I noticed you have acne," he said. "I can write a prescription for that." I thanked him and politely declined, even though I *should* have accused him of trying to mutilate my unborn children. Birth defects are just one of the documented side effects of acne medication.*

I felt embarrassed by the doc's unsolicited offer. Apparently my acne was still a prominent feature. How was I supposed to establish my reputation as a respected navy officer as a five-foot-two female with a face full of pimples?

After my tour in Virginia, the navy transferred me to Puerto Rico and then Jacksonville, Florida. In Puerto Rico my skin wasn't bad, but the acne returned in Jacksonville. I kept it under control through monthly facials (sometimes weekly) and the use of a common acne cleanser that contains high amounts of benzoyl peroxide—five times the amount found in the Proactiv line. It bleached the heck out of my towels but it was the only product that kept my acne in check.

---

*Accutane, also referred to as isotretinoin, is known to cause brain, heart, and face deformities in unborn children if taken while pregnant. After a series of lawsuits, the manufacturer withdrew Accutane from the market in 2009, but it is still available in generic form. For more information on the history and devastating side effects of this common acne medication, visit the Accutane information page at https://www.drugwatch.com /accutane.

At this point, I was nearing thirty when my skin threw me a major curveball. I had left Jacksonville to accept a Fulbright scholarship in Tunisia, another sun-soaked country on the edge of the Sahara. At the end of a day at the beach in Tunisia, I noticed a dark shadow on my upper lip. I thought it was a smudge of dirt but it wouldn't wipe off. I looked at the mirror again. What was it? I felt my stomach tighten. Is this what skin cancer looks like? Is it permanent? Will it spread?

The dark patch of skin turned out to be melasma, a common skin condition triggered by sun exposure. After researching melasma on the internet, I saw that some people drew a connection between the use of benzoyl peroxide and the onset of their melasma. I stopped using benzoyl peroxide and my melasma went away. The strange part was that my acne didn't come back either.

I spent the second part of my Fulbright studies in Scotland where, like in Tunisia, my skin was effortlessly clear. While in Scotland, I turned thirty and had a cellulite-fueled health awakening after a cliché encounter with a dressing room mirror. I cleaned up my diet and rid my apartment of toxic products. I ate wild salmon, switched to herbal tea, and started using fluoride-free toothpaste. The only time I had acne was when I broke my routine and traveled away from my little flat in St. Andrews. I remember telling a friend, "It took some work but at thirty years old, I finally figured out how to get rid of my acne."

Not yet, Melissa.

ONCE UPON A DREAM

After Scotland, I returned to the United States to live in Delray Beach, Florida, near Miami. My acne returned quickly and was the worst it had been since I lived in Newport, Rhode Island. It became so bad, I resorted to using benzoyl peroxide again, but then the melasma came back too.

I developed deep cystic welts around my mouth, along my jawline, on my forehead, down the front and back of my neck, and even inside my

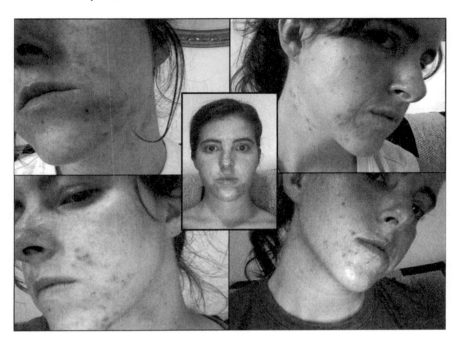

ears.* I could feel each breakout forming a week before it came to the sur-face, erupting in a tender white volcano that took another two weeks to heal. This time, with my health awakening firmly entrenched, I looked to alternative treatments to heal my skin. I used apple cider vinegar as a toner and coconut oil as a moisturizer. I coated my face in clay. I took evening primrose oil and probiotics. I went for acupuncture. I did yoga.

One night my acne was bothering me so much I couldn't sleep. I wandered downstairs to the refrigerator, desperate for relief. Lying on the couch, I gently painted my skin with yogurt. Its coldness was the only comfort I could think of for the mass of inflammation formerly known as my face. *Acne was driving me mad.* Why after all these years am I still struggling with acne? Why do I have acne even though I take meticulous care of my skin? How do people who eat nothing but junk food *not* have acne, but I do? I could not figure it out. I was defeated. Yogurt tears dripped down my face.

---

*For more of the ugly photographic evidence, see www.HiddenCauseofAcne.com/pics

I needed professional help but traditional doctors had proven useless in the past. During a required annual physical with the navy, one doctor suggested to heal my acne I should (1) stop touching my face with my hands, (2) clean telephone receivers before making phone calls, and (3) take a multivitamin. This kind of advice from physicians was insulting but typical. Clearly my skin problem was more complicated than that. They did not know me well enough to realize how ridiculous their suggestions sounded. They did not know me, or my acne story, at all.

Because of my interest in studying cellulite, I started to read about the lymphatic system and its effect on health. The lymphatic system consists of a series of nodes and vessels that circulate fluid called lymph from the tissues to the bloodstream. I decided to consult a lymph drainage specialist to see if it would help with my acne. I was fortunate to live near the Upledger Institute, one of the preeminent facilities in the world for Lymph Drainage Therapy, a light-touch therapy created by French physician Bruno Chikly. The therapist I consulted, Mya Breman, studied closely with Dr. Chikly and was a longtime practitioner at Upledger.

After each session with Mya, I noticed immediate improvement. The redness and swelling decreased overnight. Existing blemishes healed at an astounding rate. But within two to three days, my skin would return to its normal distressed state. After a few weeks of treatment, Mya suggested I take a break from our sessions until I could figure out what was causing the breakouts in the first place. Mya is a Licensed Clinical Social Worker, and at our last session, she decided to make use of her psychotherapy training to help me get to the root of the problem.

"If your acne was a cartoon character," Mya asked, "what would it look like?"

I thought the question was silly, but I followed her instructions and said the first thing that came to mind. "If my acne was a cartoon character, it would be an oil drop."

"When did this oil drop form?" she asked.

"Seventh grade," I responded.

"Are you sure it hasn't been around longer than that?" Mya asked.

In true psychotherapy style, I was soon answering questions about my deepest childhood fears. I continued to respond with the first thing that popped into my mind. I was *most* afraid of the dentist. I laughed at first, but then realized how real the fear was as a child. One year, my dentist required the extraction of four of my baby teeth. Each tooth made a cracking sound I can still hear today as it loosened from my jaw. I was seven. My mom said I was such a good little girl for the dentist and that I didn't even cry until the car ride on the way home.

I continued to ponder this unearthed childhood fear over the next few days. I thought of all the other things I hated about going to the dentist. The drooling. The scraping. The needles in places there should *not* be needles. The feeling of vulnerability while lying in the dentist's chair. The awkward fluoride trays. As a child, my dentist directed my parents to give me fluoride pills, which I later learned are the reason my teeth are slightly discolored. It's a condition called dental fluorosis and a common indicator of fluoride toxicity (Whitford 1990).

One night after my last session with Mya, I had a dream about going to the dentist. I was a small child again in the dentist's chair. There was a fluoride tray in my mouth, but this time the tray was made of glass. When the dentist tried to remove it, the tray shattered into a thousand pieces, embedding small shards of glass deep in my gums. My subconscious already knew.

I remember exactly where I was standing when the idea first struck my conscious mind. I was visiting my boyfriend's family in central Florida for Thanksgiving when I was explaining my frustration with acne to his sister, a physician. There was a glass of tap water in my hand and I was about to take a sip. I looked at the water and the idea came to me: maybe my cystic acne was caused by drinking fluoride.

I was aware that fluoride could cause acne through topical contact, a condition known as fluoroderma (Saunders 1975; Blasik and Spencer 1979). From the *Physicians' Desk Reference:* "In hypersensitive individuals, fluorides occasionally cause skin eruptions such as atopic dermatitis. . . . These hypersensitivity reactions usually disappear promptly after discontinuation of the fluoride" (1994). But I washed my face with bottled water and used nonfluoridated toothpaste. The idea did not occur to me until precisely that moment that perhaps cystic acne could be caused by fluoride *ingestion*. Case studies from the 1960s and 1970s indicate that fluoride ingestion can cause skin conditions such as dermatitis, eczema, and hives (Feltman and Kosel 1961; Shea, Gillespie, and Waldbott 1969). Could fluoride cause cystic acne too?

I did a quick internet search to see if my current residence was fluoridated. It was, and the amount was toward the upper limit of the Center for Disease Control's recommended upper guideline at the time of 1.2 milligrams per liter. The last time my skin was this bad was when I lived in Newport, Rhode Island. Do they fluoridate there? Yes. Not only that, but when I visited the Newport water municipality website, they happened to be displaying a notice to consumers informing them that a random spot test indicated they had accidentally added too much fluoride to the water—over twice the upper recommended amount— and it would take some time before it returned to recommended levels. I wondered how often they accidentally overfluoridate their population.

The whole story of my experience with acne flashed in front of me. Philadelphia, Washington, D.C., Norfolk, and Jacksonville are all fluoridated. Senegal, Puerto Rico, Tunisia, and Scotland are not. The USS *Carl Vinson* uses reverse osmosis to purify water at sea. The *Wasp* took on fluoridated water from the Norfolk Naval Station. The only time I had breakouts in Scotland was when I traveled overnight outside of St. Andrews. My toiletry bag held a small travel tube of fluoridated toothpaste.

It all made sense. My dream about the fluoride tray, my fear of dentists—my acne was caused by consuming *fluoride* and my deepest self knew it.

If anecdotal evidence is ignored in studies of acne, what do you think the medical community would say about hypotheses received through dreams and epiphanies? But the fact that the idea of fluoride-induced acne came to me this way should not be surprising. There is a long history of scientific advancements first conceived in dreams.* In his bestselling book *The Myths of Innovation,* Scott Berkun claims the experience of epiphany is misunderstood. As with the famous story of Isaac Newton discovering the law of gravity when an apple fell on his head, people mistake epiphanies for haphazard ideas when they are actually the culmination of years of careful inquiry—the piece of a puzzle that brings the full picture into view.

Berkun explains epiphanies are preceded by a long period spent understanding the problem and immersing oneself in the domain (my history with acne). Then there is a period of incubation during which the knowledge is digested and rough attempts at solutions are made (my experiments with acne treatments). Sometimes there are long pauses during incubation when progress stalls and confidence wanes (my yogurt tears).

But then, as Berkun points out, "The big insights, if they happen, occur during the depths of incubation: it's possible these pauses are minds catching up with everything they've observed" (my dream about the fluoride tray). He concludes, "When a promising idea surfaces out of the subconscious and rises into our active minds, it can feel like it came from somewhere else because we weren't aware of our subconscious thoughts while we were mowing the lawn."† Or drinking a glass of water.

Over the next few years, I put my fluoride theory to the test of experience. Unfortunately it is not a simple matter of drinking bottled water. Fluoride is insidious in the industrialized diet. It hides in food and beverages where you would never find it if you did not know to look. But whenever I had an acne flare-up, I was able to use the scientific literature to track it back to a few hours earlier when I consumed food or beverages that contained a significant amount of fluoride. This happened every time, without exception. In this way, my cystic acne

---

*For some examples, see Thomas Kuhn, *The Structure of Scientific Revolutions,* 4th ed. (Chicago: The University of Chicago Press, 2012), 122.
†See Scott Berkun, *Myths of Innovation* (Sebastapol, Canada: O'Reilly Media, 2010), 11.

served as a guide that helped me figure out how to limit my fluoride consumption and ultimately cure my chronic acne.

It was a strange coincidence, if you believe in that sort of thing, that my fluoride epiphany occurred in Polk County. Located in central Florida, Polk County is the heart of the U.S. phosphate industry. Prior to World War II, the area was known for its livestock and citrus cultivation, but after the war over a dozen phosphate plants were established there to process phosphate ore for the production of commercial fertilizer.

In the 1950s, unchecked pollution from the newly constructed phosphate plants released large quantities of fluoride into the atmosphere (Connett 2003). Raw phosphate ore is roughly 2 to 4 percent fluoride. It was absorbed by nearby vegetation, damaging 25,000 acres of citrus crops and causing mass poisoning of grazing cattle. In the words of the former president of the Polk County Cattlemen's Association, "We watched our cattle become gaunt and starved, their legs became deformed; they lost their teeth. Reproduction fell off and when a cow did have a calf, it was also affected by this malady or was a stillborn" (Linton 1970 as quoted in Connett 2003). An estimated 30,000 cattle were lost and 150,000 acres of grazing land were abandoned.

The Environmental Protection Agency (EPA) now requires "wet scrubbers" to be installed on all phosphate processing plants to capture smokestack pollution before it enters the air. *This unfiltered pollution is then barreled and sold as fluoride to our municipal water authorities for addition to public water supplies.*

Most Americans, if we think about such matters, assume the fluoride added to the public water supply is a pharmaceutical-grade fluoride like the kind used in toothpaste and mouthwash, or in government studies of the safety of fluoridation. This is not the case. Approximately 95 percent* of the fluoride used for public water fluoridation in the

*This information is available directly on the Center for Disease Control's website. See "Water Fluoridation Additives Fact Sheet" at www.cdc.gov/fluoridation/engineering/wfadditives.htm

United States is hydrofluorosilicic acid, an *unfiltered* by-product of the phosphate fertilizer industry.*

I found this fact difficult to believe until I saw it in writing on my own local municipality's annual water quality report. Next to the line where the amount of fluoride was measured within "recommended" levels is a note: "discharges from fertilizer and aluminum factories." This discharge from commercial fertilizer plants is sold to water municipalities throughout the United States and Canada, including towns near you and ones as far north as the Arctic.

A GALAXY FAR, FAR AWAY

In *The Dietary Cure for Acne,* Loren Cordain, founder of the modern paleo movement and outspoken critic of the industrialized diet, does not account for fluoride in his assessment of acne. He is so focused on the leading actors in his story of heart disease (e.g., sugar, carbs, insulin, inflammation) that he completely overlooks fluoride, a hidden but pervasive element of industrialized life.

Cordain's research philosophy provides foreshadowing that things are about to go wrong. His self-described motto, "Let the data speak for itself," is an impossibility (Cordain 2015). Data does not speak. As with intelligence analysis, scientific facts require a translator, someone to put the facts into language and tell their story to the world. The studies that uncover the facts require a designer, someone to decide which variables are important and which are not, which parameters will be accounted for and which will not. The analyst's voice cannot be removed from the data. When we fool ourselves into thinking otherwise, grave errors are to be expected.

Cordain points to the controlled human trials conducted by researchers at RMIT University in Australia as proof that a high-glycemic diet

---

*For more information on the industrial sources of fluoride used in water fluoridation, as well as issues concerning lead and arsenic contamination, see "Fluoridation Chemicals" by the Fluoride Action Network available at www.fluoridealert.org/issues /water/fluoridation-chemicals

causes acne (Smith et al. 2007a). But looking at his trump card through the lens of the fluoride theory, a different picture comes into focus. In the study, published in the *American Journal of Clinical Nutrition,* 43 males between the ages of 15 and 25 were divided into 2 groups. One group consumed a low glycemic load (LGL) diet with foods high in protein and complex carbohydrates. The other group consumed a high glycemic load (HGL) diet composed of carbohydrate-dense foods they typically ate in their regular lives. At the end of the 12-week study, researchers counted the number of acne lesions and, as expected, found a marked decrease in the group on the low-glycemic diet.

The authors of the study provide few details on the composition of the HGL and LGL diets beyond the ratio of carbs, fat, and protein, but in similar studies published a few months later by the same researchers, they include a table to illustrate the types of foods consumed by participants in each group (Smith et al. 2008a and 2008b). In addition to other foods, both groups consumed water, low-fat milk, cereals, juice, and different types of rice. Any of these foods can contain significant amounts of fluoride. But the breakfast cereals consumed by the LGL group were whole grain while the control group was given extruded corn, rice, or wheat-based cereals. As you will learn in chapter 4, extruded cereals processed in fluoridated water have been found to contain fluoride concentrations between 3.8 and 6.3 parts per million (ppm), an amount several times higher than the 0.7 ppm dose currently recommended for drinking water by dental authorities in the United States (Warren and Levy 2003). The muesli and whole oats consumed by the LGL group in the studies likely did not contain significant amounts of fluoride.

Another nuanced difference between the diets was the type of juice the participants were provided. The LGL group was given apple juice while the HGL group drank orange juice. We are not told the brands of juice but it is probable they varied widely in their fluoride content. Researchers at Tufts University measured forty-three varieties of juice and found a range of fluoride between 0.15 and 6.8 ppm (Stannard et al. 1991). Apple juice is often 100 percent juice while orange juice tends to be made from concentrate with fluoridated water. The pesticide load of the fruit also contributes to the overall fluoride content.

Furthermore, the HGL group was allowed orange-flavored soft drinks and cordial beverages, two more potential caloric sources of fluoride. Only subjects in the HGL group were allowed to eat potatoes. Were they fried and roasted—or boiled and mashed in fluoridated water? The study was conducted in the fluoridated city of Melbourne, Australia.

Looking at this study through fluoride-colored glasses, it becomes clear the research team and their randomized, controlled trials were no match for the insidious nature of a culprit like fluoride. Cordain frequently refers to the study's author as Neil Mann, a fellow professor and nutritional biochemist at RMIT University. But the primary author on all three publications cited above is listed as Robyn Smith, a postgraduate scholar funded by the National Meat Industry Training Council of Australia. I am not implying that Smith consciously influenced the study to prove a low-glycemic, high-protein diet is beneficial for reducing acne. But it is likely not a coincidence the results were good for business.

In his bestselling book *Influence,* Robert Cialdini (1984) describes the number one principle of persuasion: reciprocation. Even when given an inconsequential gift or favor, a powerful human drive kicks in and compels us to return the favor—and with interest. Sociologists have not found a single human society that does not subscribe to the rule of reciprocity, making it illogical (and unscientific) to assume the scientific results of scientific research are not skewed by the source of science funding.

Famed archaeologist Richard Leakey described the principle of reciprocity as the essence of what it means to be human. To quote Leakey, "We are human because our ancestors learned to share their food and their skills in an honored network of obligation." The power of reciprocity is so overwhelming that we are *obligated* to comply even when the gift is unwanted, let alone when it covers research costs and tuition for graduate school. Smith and Mann's studies note that Meat and Livestock Australia "had no role in data collection, data analysis, data interpretation, or submission of this article for publication" (Smith et al. 2007a). But when industry helped write the screenplay and then held casting calls for the main actors, the gorilla was not invited to audition.

To be clear, I am not arguing there are no health benefits for the paleo diet, even specifically for healing acne. As Cordain's success stories show, the paleo diet can be widely effective at reducing acne—just not for the reasons he thinks it is. To implement the diet, Cordain advises to restrict consumption of many of the potentially high-fluoride foods commonly consumed today, such as cereal, soft drinks, rice, pasta, potatoes, beans, canned fish and meats, milk, beer, wine, and other alcoholic beverages. He even recommends avoiding dates and raisins, two fruits that can cause fluoroderma flare-ups for reasons that will be explained later. (Don't worry, you won't have to eliminate all these foods from your diet to heal your acne. It will all make sense by the end of the book.) With so many items on the "do not consume" list, it is likely many paleo dieters will *almost* heal their acne. And this is exactly what their experience shows.

Cordain starts to lose his footing when he strays too far from the visible evidence he was seeing in the physical world—the lack of acne on Kitavan faces—and instead tumbles headfirst into the abstract ideas manifest predominantly in the world of scientific discourse. His book on acne is filled with the stories of, for example, IL-1 alpha (Obi-Wan) labeled as cytokine (Jedi).[*] Then there are the keratinocytes (Anakin Skywalker), which eventually become corneocytes (Darth Vader) and prevent desmosomes (Palpatine) from disintegration.[†] And of course, IGF-1 and IGFBP-3 (R2-D2 and C-3PO).[‡]

---

[*]"IL-1 alpha is a cell-to-cell messenger produced by white blood cells called monocytes. Because it is a localized hormone, it is labeled a 'cytokine' . . . " (Cordain 2006, 51).

[†]"As keratinocytes begin to turn into corneocytes, the molecular structure of the desmosomes starts to change. . . . You also know that the reason why these corneocytes stick together is because their cell-to-cell anchors (the desmosomes) fail to disintegrate properly and on time" (Cordain 2006, 40 and 59).

[‡]"One final note on the IGF-1 / IGFBP-3 story . . . the binding of IGF-1 to IGFBP-3 is not a good thing for acne sufferers because as with high glycemic load carbs, it, in effect, reduces IGFBP-3" (Cordain 2006, 50).

When asked about his research methods following the findings in Kitava, Cordain explains, "What I had to do was go back into the dermatology/medical literature and back engineer the mechanism by which a Western diet could elicit acne at the cellular level. I accomplished this by immersing myself in the salient literature to develop a hypothetical mechanism which was verified four years later by my colleague, Neil Mann" (Cordain 2011).

If instead of all that, Cordain simply limited his assessment to the phenomenon he was observing in the physical world (using the force) instead of diving into the parallel galaxy of scientific parlance (the dark side), his article would have concluded that acne vulgaris is a disease of Western civilization. Full stop. It would have brought dermatologists a giant step forward in their stated mission of identifying the ultimate cause of acne, without sending them into a wild Hoth asteroid field. (Sorry. No more *Star Wars* references. Promise.)

If we take a closer look at Otto Schaefer's "When the Eskimo Comes to Town"—the article published in 1971 that sparked Cordain's interest in studying acne as a disease of Western civilization—we see clues that fluoride played a starring role in the Inuit story. First, Schaefer makes clear the Eskimos with acne were the ones who "came to town," as the title of his article indicates. And not just any town. Eskimos with acne were seen predominantly on the streets of *larger* towns. Schaefer states, "The condition used to be unknown among Eskimos, but one can see it readily amongst teenagers on the streets of Inuvik, Frobisher Bay, and Cambridge Bay. It is far less prevalent in the smaller centers." And yes, dentists already brought their water fluoridation programs to larger towns in the Arctic at this time. Schaefer's article was written in 1971. Fluoridation began in Frobisher Bay six years earlier (Curzon and Curzon 1979). It was implemented in Inuvik in 1962.*

In addition to fluoride in the water, Eskimos were consuming

---

*The fluoridation date for Inuvik was obtained in an email to the author dated October 22, 2015, from Justin Hazenberg, Engineering Team Lead, Water and Sanitation for the Department of Municipal and Community Affairs, Government of the Northwest Territories.

fluoride hidden in other industrialized beverages. Cordain focuses on soft drinks because they contain sugar, but the imported soft drinks the Eskimos were drinking likely contained fluoride, as well, since they were mostly produced in urban centers where the water supply was fluoridated. Schaefer points out, "Many Eskimos themselves blame their pimples on the 'pop, chocolate, and candies' the youngsters consume as if addicted." In Arctic towns where drinking water was often brought in by truck, as was the case in Cambridge Bay, soft drinks offered a cheap alternative.

Another possible way Inuit societies were suddenly exposed to increased levels of fluoride was through a longstanding and seemingly innocuous legacy of colonialism: black tea. Along with sugar and tobacco, tea was a popular commodity at fur trading posts throughout Canada and is the most consumed beverage in the world, next to water. It also contains more fluoride than any other edible plant. In a 2005 study published in the *American Journal of Medicine,* Michael Whyte and his colleagues from Washington University School of Medicine measured some preparations of tea that contain fluoride at 6.5 ppm. (The maximum contaminant level currently set by the EPA for drinking water is 4 ppm.) New research outlined in the public release, "Tea Contains More Fluoride Than Once Thought" indicates the level of fluoride in tea could be even higher when using more comprehensive measuring methods (Medical College of Georgia 2010).

From countries as far spread as Chile, China, Senegal, and Jordan, to name just a few, studies show fluoride from tea consumption causes dental and skeletal fluorosis (Gomez, Weber, and Torres 1989; Cao, Zhao, and Liu 1997; Diouf et al. 1994; Fraysse et al. 1989). In Cordain, Lindeberg, and Hurtado's article on acne as a disease of Western civilization, they note the consumption of tea by the Kitavan Islanders was "close to nil," which helps explain their complete lack of acne (2002). Likewise, the Ache people in Paraguay drink yerba tea, which is derived from a species of the holly family, not the *Camellia sinensis* plant from which common black tea is produced. Yerba tea is not a significant source of fluoride.

I propose tea and other common sources of fluoride contributed to the sudden development of acne among the Eskimos in the 1960s and to the stratospheric rate of acne in our own society today—including yours.

We will return to the topic of dietary fluoride in an upcoming chapter. But first, if you associate fluoride with healthy smiles, and anti-fluoridationists with *Dr. Strangelove,* then you are likely missing a few key scenes in the fluoride story.* How could a naturally occurring mineral touted by the U.S. Center for Disease Control as one of the greatest public health achievements of the twentieth century be the underlying cause of the modern acne epidemic? You might think dentists are the main characters in that plot, but they only played a supporting role. The question is, who were they supporting? And who was supporting them?

---

*_Dr. Strangelove_ is a 1964 film that old people point to as evidence that people who disagree with them about fluoride are conspiracy theorists. It might be peer-reviewed, but I'm not sure because it seems anecdotal and profluoridationists supposedly aren't into that sort of thing. You can view the scene in question at www.HiddenCauseofAcne .com/Strangelove.

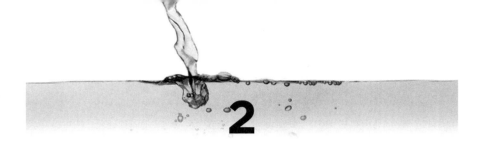

2

F: The Invisible Element behind the Modern Acne Epidemic

It started as an observation, that soon took the shape of an idea. It ended, five decades later, as a scientific revolution that shot dentistry into the forefront of preventive medicine. This is the story of how dental science discovered—and ultimately proved to the world—that fluoride, a mineral found in rocks and soil, prevents tooth decay. Although dental caries remains a public health worry, it is no longer the unbridled problem it once was, thanks to fluoride.

NATIONAL INSTITUTE OF
DENTAL AND CRANIOFACIAL RESEARCH,
FROM "THE STORY OF FLUORIDATION"

HOW THE WEST WAS WON

The full story of fluoridation cannot be contained in a book, let alone a single chapter, but even in the official version—such as the one told as of February 15, 2017, on the website of the National Institute of Dental and Craniofacial Research (NIDCR)—it is not difficult to see the heart of a deeper story beating just beneath the surface.

According to the official narrative, the story of fluoridation begins with a young dentist who literally rides west and rescues local children from unsightly smiles. I will summarize this version of the story using much of their same wording.* See if you can spy any hidden story lines, including the big hairy gorilla who struts across the stage halfway through.

Frederick McKay was a young dental school graduate who left Pennsylvania to open a dental practice in Colorado Springs. When McKay arrived in Colorado, he was astounded to find scores of local citizens with grotesque brown stains on their teeth. He searched in vain for information on the bizarre disorder, but there was a lack of interest among most area dentists. Local residents blamed the problem on any number of strange factors. McKay took up the gauntlet and researched the disorder himself, discovering that teeth afflicted with the brown stain were surprisingly and inexplicably resistant to decay.

McKay didn't know what was causing the brown stain, but that changed when he was contacted by H. V. Churchill, the chief chemist at the Aluminum Company of America (Alcoa). Churchill, who had spent the past few years refuting claims that aluminum was poisonous, conducted a special analysis of the water in Bauxite, a company town owned by Alcoa. (The name of the city was derived from its large reserve of bauxite, a natural material used in the manufacturing of aluminum.) The chemist's analysis identified fluoride as the culprit for the brown stains on children's teeth, and he kindly offered "that we may cooperate in an attempt to discover what part 'fluorine' may play in the matter."

Government research on fluoride and its effect on tooth enamel began in earnest. The architect of these first fluoride studies was H. Trendley Dean, head of the Dental Hygiene Unit at the National Institute of Health. Dean made the critical discovery that fluoride levels up to 1 ppm in drinking water do not cause enamel fluorosis in most

---

*To read the full story as described on the NIDCR website, visit www.HiddenCauseofAcne.com/resources

people. He recalled from McKay's studies that mottled tooth enamel is unusually resistant to decay and he wondered if adding fluoride to drinking water would help fight cavities. This hypothesis, Dean told his colleagues, would need to be tested. Dean got his wish in 1945 when Grand Rapids, Michigan, became the first city in the world to fluoridate its drinking water.

The Grand Rapids water fluoridation study was originally sponsored by the U.S. Surgeon General, but was taken over by the National Institute of Dental Research shortly after its inception in 1948, with Dean as the new institute's director. The results of Dean's fifteen-year study in Grand Rapids were astounding. Cavities dropped by more than 60 percent after fluoride was added, leading to water fluoridation projects throughout the country that currently benefit over 200 million Americans. McKay, Dean, and the others helped to transform dentistry into a prevention-oriented profession. Their drive, in the face of overwhelming adversity, is no less than a remarkable feat of science—an achievement ranking with the other great preventive health measures of our century.

A Hollywood fraternity of preteen dental groupies could not have imagined a better plot. There's a young altruistic dentist hero. Confused townspeople. Vulnerable children. There's a big mystery, then it's solved. And in the end, a wise government dentist brings health and happiness to millions of people around the globe, establishing American dentistry at the forefront of preventive medicine. If you look closely, however, you'll see clues even the NIDCR story does not hide. The deeper story of fluoridation is not about rescuing people from cavities—it is about *pollution.*

Reading the story above with a skeptical twenty-first-century eye, one might be suspicious of the presence of the Alcoa chemist whose bit part was the discovery that fluoride was responsible for the browning of children's teeth. Why was Alcoa studying fluoride, and why was their chief chemist so eager to cooperate with dentists?

One of the most common elements in the Earth's crust, fluoride is also the most reactive. Because of its high reactivity, fluoride is not found on its own in nature but is bound with common metals and minerals such as bauxite and phosphate. In addition, fluoride has the prized ability of lowering the melting point of metals, making it a bedrock of key manufacturing processes. This explains why fluoride is a by-product of so many industries, from aluminum plants and phosphate processors to steel mills, coal burning operations, and brick and tile manufacturers.

America has largely forgotten that fluoride is a major pollutant, but a 1972 handbook from the U.S. Department of Agriculture entitled "Air Pollutants Affecting the Performance of Domestic Animals" states, "Airborne fluorides have caused more worldwide damage to domestic animals than any other air pollutant." In 1983, Leonard Weinstein, a Cornell professor and international authority on the effect of fluorides in plants, noted, "Certainly, there has been more litigation on alleged damage to agriculture by fluoride than all other pollutants combined" (as quoted in Bryson 2011, 197). To reduce their vulnerability to lawsuits from fluoride pollution, corporations were all too willing to work closely with dentists studying fluoride so they could keep an eye on the science and help direct their research.

In 1913, Alcoa leaders took this strategy a step further when they created the Mellon Institute of Industrial Research at the University of Pittsburgh. Alcoa-funded researchers at the Mellon Institute were the first to make a public proposal to add fluoride to the water supply (Bryson 2011). Similarly, the Kettering Laboratory of Applied Physiology at the University of Cincinnati was established in 1930 by other corporations with a self-interest in proving the safety of fluoride, including DuPont and General Motors. By 1931, the majority of the Kettering Laboratory's research focused on fluoride. Researchers from Kettering spent their careers refuting studies that revealed the dangers of fluoride exposure. When their own studies indicated fluoride has severe health consequences, the results were never published and were literally hidden in the basement.*

What about Dean's fifteen-year experiment in Grand Rapids that proved fluoridation safe and effective? The flaws are difficult to hide even from our little layman brains. To give just one obvious example, the study was designed to have a control city so researchers could compare the long-term effects of fluoridation in Grand Rapids with the nonfluoridated city of Muskegon, Michigan. But only five years into the fifteen-year study, fluoride was added to the public water supply in Muskegon too (Arnold et al. 1956). This did not hinder the researchers, though, and they confidently concluded that fluoride caused the drop in dental decay.

Without a control city, researchers measuring the rate of dental decay in fluoridated Grand Rapids did not see that the rate of dental decay decreased in nonfluoridated cities as well. Statistical analysis of data from the World Health Organization clearly shows the decline in tooth decay occurred equally in nonfluoridated cities throughout the Western world as nutrition improved following the Depression Era (Connett 2012g).

The Grand Rapids study is littered with these types of blatant inadequacies. Hubert Arnold, a statistician from the University of California at Davis, used the fluoridation trials to demonstrate poor statistical analysis to his students. According to Arnold, the studies "are especially rich in fallacies, improper design, invalid use of statistical methods, omissions of contrary data, and just plain muddleheadedness and hebetude" (Arnold to Newbrun as quoted in Connett 2010, 51).

In June 2015, the Cochrane Group, a U.K.-based organization

---

*For example, when a metal company lost a lawsuit in 1957 involving fluoride's effect on soft tissue, Kettering researchers were instructed to find evidence to refute future claims. Instead, their 1958 study involving forty-two beagle dogs showed fluoride, when inhaled, quickly enters the bloodstream and causes damage to lungs and lymph nodes. Industry lawyers were sent copies of the study, but it was hidden from the public until investigative journalist Christopher Bryson combed through the basement archives of the old Kettering Laboratory at the University of Cincinnati decades later (Bryson 2011, 188).

described in *Newsweek* as "the gold standard of scientific rigor in assessing effectiveness of public health policies," reviewed every official study they could locate on fluoridation and found that in 97 percent, the risk of bias was high (Main 2015a; Zipporah et al. 2015). The Cochrane review concluded there is very little evidence on the effectiveness of water fluoridation for the prevention of dental decay.

Far from "proving to the world" the benefits of fluoridation, as the NIDCR narrative states, most developed countries do not consume artificially fluoridated water, including approximately 97 percent of western Europe.* When Sweden's Nobel Prize–winning scientist, pharmacologist Dr. Arvid Carlsson, investigated the proposal of water fluoridation for his country, he soon became an outspoken critic of the practice. "Fluoridation is against all principles of modern pharmacology," Carlsson concluded. "Those nations that are using it should feel ashamed of themselves. It's against science" (Carlsson 2005). Even without fluoridation, Sweden experienced the same decline in tooth decay as was observed in heavily fluoridated countries like the United States (Connett 2012g).

Industry did not rely solely on biased and naive researchers to advance their interests in fluoride—there were lawyers involved as well. Following a spike in industrial fluoride pollution during World War II, the threat of litigation was overwhelming. "Soon we had claims and lawsuits around aluminum smelters from coast to coast," explained Alcoa's leading fluoride litigator, Frank Seamans (1983 as quoted in Bryson 2011, 102).

Seamans responded to the crisis by forming a self-described "Fluorine Lawyers Committee" with fluoride litigators collaborating from U.S. Steel, Monsanto Chemical, the Tennessee Valley Authority, and several other large corporations vulnerable to fluoride pollution lawsuits. The Fluorine Lawyers Committee met regularly to strategize

---

*To view the reasoning in their own words, see "Statements from European Health, Water, and Environment Authorities on Water Fluoridation" at www.fluoridealert.org /content/europe-statements. Be sure to click the red "Source" link next to each country to view the official response directly from the relevant authority.

ways to defuse "the fluoride problem," and they played a strong role in directing fluoride research.*

The full effect of industry interest on public fluoridation policy in the United States is impossible to quantify. The corporations most affected by fluoride pollution were the most powerful companies in the world, and vital partners with U.S. military and government officials throughout the world wars. When the U.S. Public Health Service prematurely endorsed public water fluoridation in 1950—ten years *before* the conclusion of Dean's fluoridation trial in Grand Rapids—perhaps it should not have come as a surprise. The decision was made under the leadership of Oscar R. Ewing, who was designated as head of the Federal Security Agency over the Public Health Service in 1947. Ewing was a longtime Alcoa lawyer and performed legal work for Alcoa in Washington until 1945.

IN FLUORIDE WE TRUST

For those who are aware of the dirty history of public water fluoridation, it can be hard to believe the practice is still championed today. If the supporting science is overwhelmingly flawed, why does the practice persist? Biased dentists and callous lawyers could not accomplish such an impressive feat on their own. For that, industry had to bring in the sorcerers.

What the official story of fluoride lacks in sophistication and scientific rigor, it makes up for in marketing magic. In his 2006 book *Primal Branding: Create Zealots for Your Brand, Your Company, and Your Future,* Forbes branding expert Patrick Hanlon explains that "brands

---

*The influence of industry lawyers on fluoride research was blatant. One internal document from Seamans to other members of the Fluorine Lawyers Committee dated April 16, 1957, and labeled "research re human beings" includes an attachment Seamans sent to medical directors at Kettering "in which an attempt is made to more specifically advise just what the lawyers group wishes them to do" (Seamans to Robert Kehoe, Kettering Files, file 17, box 42, quoted in Bryson 2011, 188).

are belief systems." He identifies seven primal branding elements that inspire fans to rabid addiction: the creation story, the leader, the creed, rituals, icons, sacred words, and pagans. Hanlon refers to these seven factors as primal code. When the seven elements of the primal code are firmly in place, a brand resonates deep in the public psyche, creating "a belief system and products and services that people can believe in" (Hanlon 2006, 6). This is how successful brands become a meaningful part of our culture.

Hanlon describes a brand as any product, service, organization, social cause, religion, movement, or other entity searching for popular appeal. In this sense, fluoridation is a brand, and it expertly incorporates every element of the primal branding message. By dissecting the official story of fluoridation from a branding perspective, we see why it has proven resistant to change in the face of sound contradictory science. It is because fluoridation is not a science. It is a religion.

Primal Branding Element #1: The Creation Story

Hanlon describes the creation story as "the foundation of trust" for a new belief system, fulfilling an innate desire to know how we came to be. It often involves a mythic quest or an against-all-odds pursuit, and it is the crucial first step that provides answers to why people should care about you, or your product or service. The NIDCR makes clear their story of fluoridation is also the story of the establishment of the National Institute of Dental Research (the predecessor to the NIDCR), which was founded during the early years of the Grand Rapids experiment. Fluoridation was not just a great discovery dentists claim to have made—it is the creation story for the entire U.S. dental system.

Primal Branding Element #2: The Leader

"All successful belief systems have a person who is the catalyst, the risk taker, the visionary," Hanlon writes. In the story of fluoridation, the leading figure is H. Trendley Dean. Dean was the first director of the National Institute of Dental Research, meaning that in addition to being "the father of fluoridation," he is also the father of government institutionalized dentistry in the United States. Dean was selected for this position specifically because of his work with fluoridation. To question fluoridation is to undermine modern dentistry's founding father.

Primal Branding Element #3: The Creed

The creed is the singular notion a brand wants people to believe. It is based on a set of core principles that define a company's mission and explains who they are and why they exist. With the story of fluoridation, dentists brand themselves as heroes rescuing a helpless population from dental decay. To underline this notion, they repeat mantras such as "fluoride is safe and effective" and "fluoridation is one of the greatest public health achievements of the twentieth century" with blind faith in the institutionalized belief system from which such claims originated.

Primal Branding Element #4: Sacred Words

"All belief systems come with a set of specialized words that must be learned before people can belong," Hanlon states. The medical community is infamous for such jargon. For example, while nondentists speak of cavities and tooth decay, dentists use the term "dental caries." *Caries* is simply the Latin word for "rottenness," but peer-reviewed publications on the rate of "dental rottenness" would not sound quite as professional. Those who buy in to a brand use sacred words as protection for the group's ideals, since they assume members of the group are the only ones who can speak the language. For example, early in the fluoridation effort, the American Dental Association (ADA) advised dentists that fluoridation "should not be submitted to the voters, who cannot possibly sift through and comprehend the scientific evidence" (Bryson 2011).

Primal Branding Element #5: Rituals

Rituals are repeated interactions consumers have with a brand. They are touch points that solidify the brand in the lives of its supporters and highlight the brand's meaning and relevance. The incorporation of both daily and intermittent rituals anchors the fluoride brand firmly in American culture. Adding fluoride to toothpaste brought the twice-daily ritual of fluoride into our homes. We are also chided to visit the dentist twice per year to soak our teeth in fluoride. Marketers now recognize that internal branding is also fundamental to a brand's success. For dentists, the use of fluoride trays is a daily ritual they perform on their patients, while an example of an annual ritual is the celebration of the birth of fluoridation.*

Primal Branding Element #6: Icons

Hanlon describes icons as "quick concentrations of meaning that cause your brand identity and brand values to spontaneously resonate." Often icons are visual, but they can be any sensory trigger that summons the basic substance of the brand. The fluoride logo currently displayed on the homepage for the American Dental Association is a perfect example. Next to a tagline that reads "Fluoride to the rescue!" is a sparkly white tooth with a *T* superhero emblem on its chest (notice they didn't use an *F*). Flexing its muscular arms, the tooth is surrounded by little bubbles of sodium fluoride indicated by the periodic symbols F and Na. The entire logo, of course, is red, white, and blue. The icons for fluoridation are not always so cartoonish. A tube of toothpaste is an iconic symbol of fluoride's pervasiveness in American culture. The dentist's waiting room with its requisite magazines, even the dentist's chair—these are icons that evoke the notion of dental authority and reinforce the brand's message of dentist as hero.

Primal Branding Element #7: Pagans and Nonbelievers

Pagans are the final element in the primal marketing code. "Defining your pagans is important in defining who you are," Hanlon writes. Recent examples are 7UP declaring itself "the uncola" and Taco Bell urging its

---

*As I wrote this paragraph on September 11, 2015, dentists were attending the Seventieth Anniversary Fluoridation Celebration and Symposium in Chicago.

audience to "think outside the bun." Believers serve both as brand evangelists and defenders. When the brand is threatened, they protect it as if they are the ones under attack. Believers who express doubt are excommunicated and exiled to the opposing camp. This explains why profluoridationists fixate on the caricature of antifluoride conspiracy theorists depicted in *Dr. Strangelove,* and why decades of contradictory research barely made a dent in fluoride's superhero status. By pushing against a fanatical belief system, opponents unwittingly make it stronger.

When fluoridation is viewed as a belief system, not a science, it becomes apparent why the practice continues today. Successful brands "fulfill genuine pieces of the human psyche," Hanlon writes. "Believing is belonging."

Questioning the fluoride brand inherently translates as an attack on the entire U.S. dental culture. Its creation story, leader, creed, sacred words, rituals, icons, and pagans are all wrapped up in the story of fluoridation. H. Trendley Dean could not have been a shoddy researcher; he was the founding father. Fluoridation could not have been a ploy by fluoride polluters; it is the NIDCR's reason for existence. How can fluoride be bad for your health if the majority of the U.S. population drinks eight glasses a day?

Sigmund Freud himself could not have conceived of a more brilliant psychological strategy to inculcate American minds with the notion that it is a good idea to put toxic waste from aluminum plants directly into the water supply—but his nephew could.

It is not a coincidence that one of the most controversial public health practices of the twenty-first century is also one of the most successful brands in modern history. All seven pieces of the primal marketing code did not fall into place by happenstance. It was by design. The designer was Edward Bernays, who earned his title as the "Father of Public Relations" by combining insights from the burgeoning field of crowd psychology with ideas from psychoanalysis as developed by his uncle, Sigmund Freud.

Bernays's most famous campaign involved staging a group of women suffragists to march in the Easter parade in New York City holding lit cigarettes in the air as "torches of freedom." Women were previously banned from smoking in public outside of designated areas, but by turning smoking into a women's suffragist issue, the publicity from Bernays's campaign helped tobacco companies break a social taboo that was impeding their entry into a mainstream market.

Bernays's work on fluoridation is less well known but even more ingenious. Again, his efforts in New York City provide a brilliant example of his campaign tactics. "If New York City accepts an idea, the other states will accept the idea too," he told journalist Christopher Bryson, author of *The Fluoride Deception,* in a 1993 interview. The fluoridation debate raged in New York in the early 1960s and was described by the *New York Times* as "one of the most contentious issues of the Cold War" (Blumenthal 2015). The antifluoridation movement had successfully stalled fluoridation for several years and was led by leading physicians such as Simon Beisler, former president of the American Urological Association, and Fred Squier Dunn, chief of the Dental Department at the renowned Lenox Hill Hospital in Manhattan.

In a letter written to Leona Baumgartner, the New York Health Commissioner, Bernays describes the public relations strategy he helped implement for fluoridation. In the letter, he counsels the health commissioner to write to television executives at NBC and CBS and tell them debating fluoridation "is like presenting two sides for anti-Catholicism or anti-Semitism and therefore not in the public interest." He warns her not to ask them to act in a specific way, but to generally plant the idea in their minds that fluoridation should not be debated. "This might lead to a revision of the whole policy of what shall and shall not be considered controversial," Bernays predicts (Bernays to Baumgartner 1960 as quoted in Bryson 2011, 161).

The campaign included sending government letters to influential newspaper editors and even publishers of dictionaries and encyclopedias. The letters were not to argue for fluoridation or address concerns of critics; their purpose was to leverage government influence to dominate the fluoridation narrative and marginalize opposition. In this way, pro-fluoridationists manipulated the human tendency to defer to authority sources, such as doctors, dictionaries, and the daily news. Bernays referred to this technique as the *engineering of consent,* which relies on *third-party authorities* to give credence to a brand or product. "You can get practically any idea accepted," Bernays told Bryson (2011, 159). "If doctors are in favor, the public is willing to accept it, because a doctor is an authority to most people, regardless of how much he knows, or doesn't know. . . . By the law of averages, you can usually find an individual in any field who will be willing to accept new ideas."

In his seminal book *Propaganda,* Bernays describes his philosophy behind the engineering of consent further. "Those who manipulate this unseen mechanism of society constitute an invisible government which is the true ruling power of our country," he writes. "It is they who pull the wires which control the public mind" (1928, 38).

Bernays spent his retirement in penance supporting antismoking campaigns, claiming he would have refused to work with the tobacco industry if he knew of the negative health effects of cigarettes earlier. He seems not to have realized that even while helping to pull the strings, he was part of the public mind that was being controlled.

REDCOATS AND REBELS

Once a belief system is manifest in government institutions, it becomes deeply entrenched in a culture and, like a mastodon in quicksand, nearly impossible to budge. It's not that present-day government officials and dentists are evil beings who knowingly poison the population and the planet to protect their precious fluoridation scheme. They are regular people who see what they expect to see and feel safe when siding with the majority and the status quo.

The longer a brand is established, the more layered it becomes as complementary entities grow around it and reinforce the belief structure. These patrons can be offshoots of the brand or entirely separate entities that gravitate to the brand because they share a common interest. In the story of fluoridation, we find both types.

One such patron is the dental hygiene industry. Fluoridated toothpaste is a dream product for an entrepreneur. It must be repurchased on a regular and frequent basis, it has a price point that makes it both accessible to the masses and massively profitable, and it is endorsed by third-party authorities as an indispensable part of daily life for everyone, everywhere—not just once a day, but two times or more.*

Proctor & Gamble (P&G) set out to dominate the fluoride toothpaste market when it launched the Crest brand in the 1950s, originally marketed under the unfortunate name Fluoristan. Renamed as Crest with Fluoristan, the new line was unveiled with an ad campaign featuring Norman Rockwell paintings of gleeful children proudly waving their dental checkup cards. The campaign tagline, "Look, Mom—no cavities!" raised concerns at the time about truth in advertising. At a congressional hearing in 1958, the assistant secretary for the American Dental Association's (ADA) Counsel on Dental Therapeutics claimed the ads were "at best both a gross exaggeration and a misleading distortion" (McDonough and Egolf 2002, 420).

Just two years later (the same year Bernays started his fluoridation campaign for the New York Health Commissioner), the ADA suddenly changed its mind about Crest and selected it as the first and only toothpaste to receive the ADA seal of approval. Within one year of the announcement, Crest more than doubled its share of the toothpaste market. As an added benefit, future truth-in-advertising complaints were circumvented simply by referring to the ADA endorsement as proof that Crest fights cavities.

Now that Crest was widely profitable, P&G took over the marketing of fluoride where Bernays's campaign left off. Until the 1980s,

---

*For an enlightening account of how marketers hooked the world on foamy mint toothpaste, see Charles Duhigg, *The Power of Habit: Why We Do What We Do in Life and Business* (New York: Random House, 2012), 31–37.

P&G spent more money on advertising for Crest than any other brand in its extensive lineup, including Tide laundry detergent, Ivory soap, and Pampers diapers (McDonough and Egolf 2002). By the end of the twentieth century, the company was spending upwards of $90 million *per year* on advertising for Crest products, ensuring the official story of fluoride remained deeply instilled in the American psyche.

Financial proceeds from fluoridated products continue to find their way back to government supporters through grants and donations, strategic partnerships, and industry-sponsored nonprofit organizations.* In 2014, Crest toothpaste alone generated over $380 million in sales (Statista n.d.).

Other patrons of fluoridation are not as overt. In November 2007, Cristin Kearns, a dental administrator for Kaiser Permanente's Dental Care Program, attended a conference in Seattle intended to educate dentists on the links between diabetes and gum disease. She was suspicious when the keynote speaker insisted "there is no research to support that sugar causes chronic disease." Her experience working in low-income dental clinics in Denver told her otherwise.

Kearns suspected the sugar industry might be manipulating the nutritional advice dental professionals like herself were receiving. A Google search for "International Sugar Research Foundation" and "archives" led her to a neglected trove of firsthand evidence of the subversive role the sugar industry had long been playing in dental research. The University of Illinois librarian who archived the files from a bankrupt sugar company thought they mostly documented the impact of the beet sugar industry on farm labor, but as Kearns soon realized, they documented much more than that.

---

*One such group is Friends of NIDCR, a nonprofit organization whose mission is "to educate the public and key decision makers about the importance of investing in the NIDCR." To return the sentiment, at their annual conference in Washington, D.C., Friends of NIDCR hosts a roundtable discussion whose mission is "to drive awareness amongst the oral health community of the role that industry plays in the success of Pulic/Private Partnerships (PPPs)." The first roundtable was chaired by Dr. J. Leslie Winston, scientific relations director at Proctor & Gamble.

The cache of internal documents, which Kearns quit her job to study, revealed the sugar industry's shockingly close ties with the National Institute of Dental Research (NIDR) in the 1960s and 1970s while it was building the National Caries Program, an initiative implemented under President Nixon in 1971 with the goal of ending dental decay in a decade.

In March 2015, Kearns, now a postdoctoral fellow at the University of California–San Francisco (UCSF), published a paper with her findings in the peer-reviewed journal *PLoS Medicine*. Along with her two coauthors, Kearns revealed the NIDR steering committee tasked with prioritizing research initiatives for dental decay was composed almost entirely of personnel from the International Sugar Research Foundation's (ISRF) Scientific Advisory Board, whose stated purpose was "to discover effective means of controlling tooth decay by methods other than restricting carbohydrate intake" (Kearns, Glantz, and Schmidt 2015). The sugar industry needed dentists to focus on a way to strengthen teeth so they would be distracted from identifying the true cause of dental decay—which is not a lack of fluoride, but an excess of sugar.

As with the fluoride polluters decades before, the sugar industry encouraged fluoride as a dental treatment to hide evidence of its own vulnerability. The internal documents reveal industry scientists were well aware of sugar's leading role in dental decay as early as 1950, and they promoted programs on enzymes, dental vaccines, and fluoride in an effort to deflect attention from sugar as the culprit.

When the National Caries Program submitted their omnibus request for contracts in 1971, which set the precedent for the direction dental research would take for the years ahead, the authors of the request copied verbatim or closely paraphrased 78 percent of a report the sugar industry submitted to the NIDR two years earlier (Kearns, Glantz, and Schmidt 2015).

While the patrons of fluoridation are behemoth billion-dollar juggernauts, the pagans are quite the opposite: individuals who, through circumstance, became aware of the inaccuracies, inadequacies, and injustices of the fluoridation story and decided to do something about it. They have limited financial backing, political influence, or media access and thus are easily dismissed, crucified, or ignored altogether. Much of their efforts have been bulldozed by the fluoride faithful who cling to the creed that "fluoridation is safe and effective" and block out all evidence to the contrary. Profluoridationists want to believe (and want you to believe) that qualified critics of fluoridation do not exist, but the following vignettes offer a glimpse of some of the protagonists on the other side of the fluoridation story through the years.

Kaj Roholm

Cryolite mines in Denmark made the country an early testbed for fluoride pollution. Roholm, the Deputy Health Commissioner of Copenhagen, authored the 1937 tome *Fluoride Intoxication,* a monumental study of the toxic effects of fluoride, including a forty-page bibliography with 893 references to scientific articles. Roholm noted the amount of fluoride recommended in the United States to prevent tooth decay was close to the toxic limit and warned, "The particular danger in the therapeutic use of fluorine compounds is the development of a chronic intoxication." Recognized as the world's leading expert on fluoride toxicity, Roholm was unable to defend his work from the inevitable harsh criticism it received in the United States during the early fluoridation era due to his untimely death from cancer in 1948.

George Waldbott

After graduating from medical school in Germany, Waldbott accepted a residency in Michigan where he embarked on a pioneering career in the study and treatment of allergic diseases. Beginning in the 1950s, he published numerous research papers that indicated a significant portion of the population is hypersensitive to fluoride. He spent the rest of his life advocating against public water fluoridation, founding the International Society for Fluoride Research and its quarterly journal, *Fluoride.* Described as an "eminent" allergist even by his critics (Prival 1972), official studies were never attempted to refute his findings.

Phyllis Mullenix

After receiving her doctorate in pharmacology, Mullenix worked at Johns Hopkins School of Public Health and then Harvard Medical School until she was selected to establish the toxicology department at the Forsyth Dental Center in Boston in 1983, the first toxicology department in any dental institution in the world. After her supervisor encouraged her to study fluoride, she was surprised when the science indicated fluoride is a neurotoxin. She was even more surprised when health officials ignored her research and cut off her funding. She was then fired from her position at Forsyth (Mullenix 2000).

John Colquhoun

An ardent fluoridation advocate, Colquhoun was chairman of New Zealand's Fluoridation Promotion Committee when research on fluoride started to raise questions in his mind about its safety and effectiveness. Colquhoun reversed his stance on fluoride in the early 1980s, a move that cost him his prestigious position as the Principal Dental Officer of Auckland, the country's largest city. In 1991, he became a board member of the International Society of Fluoride Research, as well as the editor of its journal *Fluoride*. Colquhoun outlined his reasons for opposing fluoridation in a 1997 journal article published in *Perspectives in Biology and Medicine* by Johns Hopkins University Press.

William Marcus

A leading toxicologist at the EPA's Office of Drinking Water, Marcus was fired in 1992 after raising health concerns about fluoride. He filed a lawsuit under the Whistleblower Protection Act and, after a fierce two-year court battle, prevailed on every count. He was reinstated to his job at the EPA but continued to experience harassment, later filing and winning a second hearing over his hostile work environment.

Court evidence revealed collusion between EPA managers and numerous chemical companies.* Marcus's health concerns over fluoride were never addressed in EPA policy.

Hardy Limeback

Former president of the Canadian Association for Dental Research, Limeback headed the Department of Preventive Dentistry at the University of Toronto. After publishing numerous papers on the benefits of fluoridation and serving as a consultant on fluoride to the Canadian Dental Association, Limeback, who also has a doctorate in collagen biochemistry, changed his position on fluoridation in the 1990s after examining the effect of ingested fluorides on bone development (2000). He was subsequently passed over by Canadian health officials from participating in future fluoridation reviews.

William Hirzy

A senior scientist at the EPA's Office of Pollution Prevention and Toxics, Hirzy was also President of the EPA Headquarters Union. His attention turned to fluoride in 1985 when the EPA was revising its drinking water standard for fluoride. An employee complained to the union that he was being coerced to write an assessment he did not support. For the rest of his career, Hirzy represented 1,500 EPA professionals in the union's opposition to fluoridation. He even testified before the U.S. Senate on behalf of the union in June 2000 regarding the union's rejection of public water fluoridation. You can view a video of Hirzy's Senate testimony at www.HiddenCauseofAcne.com/Hirzy.

Paul Connett

With degrees from Cambridge and Dartmouth, Connett was a professor of chemistry and toxicology for twenty-three years at St. Lawrence

---

*For a 1995 interview with William Marcus, visit http://fluoridealert.org/content /marcus-interview

University before retiring to found the Fluoride Action Network (FAN) in May 2000, a nonprofit organization dedicated to raising awareness of the health effects of fluoride exposure. Connett and the FAN team gather the latest news and research on fluoride, provide input to policy makers, and support local antifluoridation campaigners. (The research gathered on FAN's extensive website, fluoridealert.org, was invaluable in healing my acne.)

These are just a few of the perfectly credentialed scientists whose voices have been marginalized by fluoridation proponents. I am tempted to continue with other examples because their stories are important, but they always have the same plot. Nonbelievers suggest fluoridation has negative health effects and call for research and caution, while dentists point to a lack of evidence and cite the creed—"more than [x] years of scientific research has consistently shown that an optimal level of fluoride in community water is safe and effective."*

If this is the first time you are learning about the underground story of fluoridation, you might be feeling disheartened, angry, powerless, or in a state of disbelief. With fluoridation so deeply entrenched in American culture, how can individuals like you and me ever hope to change it?

Not to worry. There is a plan.† In the meantime, to heal your acne, you do not need to change anything that is not already well within your reach to change. You just need to turn the page.

---

*This phrase was taken directly from the ADA webpage on fluoridation on September 19, 2015, at www.ada.org/en/public-programs/advocating-for-the-public /fluoride-and-fluoridation
†See the appendix at the end of this book. Also, www.HiddenCauseofAcne.com/STOP

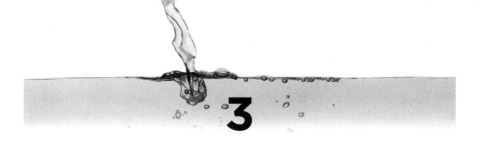

3

Rethinking the Cause of Your Acne

LET'S RECAP. Eskimos start experiencing acne when they move to town. Dermatologists develop a drug addiction. Native Kitavans never get acne. The Ache don't either. Paleo godfather *almost* cures acne. Dentists create a fluoride cult. Avoiding fluoride cures my acne. That brings us to the current point in our story. Here is where your part comes in.

TALES FROM GOTHAM CITY

After my fluoride epiphany in 2008, I tested my fluoride hypothesis on my own skin so many times the results were undeniable, even for family members who originally thought I was crazy when I told them tap water makes my skin break out (be forewarned, family members tend to do that). It took a few years for me to figure out how to reduce my exposure enough to heal my chronic acne for good, but by 2010 my breakouts were nonexistent.

Along the way, I was sharing my experience with fluoride on a small health blog I started writing, and almost immediately some of the people who read my posts on acne said they also started noticing breakouts from fluoride. It was strange. I assumed fluoride-induced acne was an obscure condition. I had never heard of it before. None of the experts

I consulted over the years mentioned it. The scientific literature was sparse. Even the internet didn't seem to know much about it.

In 2011, I posted a free guide on my site explaining the basics of fluoride and acne. Keep in mind, most people who visited the site did so because of their interest in cellulite, not acne. I typically received only a couple hundred visitors per day, and my bounce rate (the amount of people who leave without looking around) was consistently close to 70 percent. That's not good. Even my most popular acne post only received a handful of views per day, if any. However, despite my total lack of blogging skills, I started to receive success stories from other people who cured their cystic acne by avoiding fluoride.

It should have been highly improbable that someone suffering from acne would (1) find my website, (2) read my guide, (3) implement my recommendations, (4) heal their acne, and (5) come back to tell me about it. I did some quick math. If I had already heard from this many people with fluoride-induced acne, how many more of us were out there?

Over the next few years, in addition to the testimonials coming in from visitors to my website, I caught glimpses of the gorilla around town more and more. A man on the plane with deep welts down his chin and neck. A young woman at work with heavy makeup trying to hide cysts along her jawline.

The gorilla was hanging out all over the online acne forums too. The experts all pinky swore never ever to read health information on the internet, *especially* the comments and forums. But intelligence analysts and other trained investigators know, sometimes your best source for intel is the man on the street. Once you know that fluoride-induced acne is a thing, it's not difficult to see it hiding in the comments people leave on various health and beauty websites. Because of copyright restrictions, I won't include them here, but I will link to a few examples at www.HiddenCauseofAcne.com/clues so you know what I am talking about.

Before I am written up by the science hall monitors, I realize these examples are anecdotal (but not in the pejorative sense). None of the commenters suspect fluoride as the cause of their acne, and even if they did, their suspicions would likely be speculative. And yes, with the gazillions of comments on the internet, you could likely find at least a couple to support the theory that acne is caused by rainbow kryptonite. These are all valid points. I am not trying to *prove* fluoroderma exists by cherry picking anecdotal evidence from the internet. These accounts are simply a few real-world *illustrations* that I am incorporating into my larger proposition that fluoride-induced acne is not an uncommon condition— and that we will only recognize it once we know to look. My aim with this book is to encourage other people, like you, to start looking.

Anecdotal has become a curse word in the modern medical world, but the experiences of individuals like you and me have their place in scientific inquiry. The Cambridge dictionary defines *anecdotal* information as "not based on facts or careful study." According to Merriam-Webster, it means "based on or consisting of reports or observations of usually unscientific observers." But the etymology of the word suggests something different.

The word *anecdotal* goes back to the ancient Greek idea of *anekdota,* from *an,* "not," and *ekdota,* "published." The meaning of *anecdotal* started to change when Procopius, the last major historian of the ancient world, used it as the title of his scandalous account of the venal and salacious private lives of Roman emperor Justinian and his wife, Theodora. (See what Procopius did there? He took a word that meant *unpublished* and he published it. That Procopius!) His book, based on court gossip, gave the word *anecdotal* a sense of "revelation of secrets," which then degraded in English into "brief, amusing stories" and finally "dubious support of a generalized claim," as anecdotal evidence is currently described on Wikipedia.

But an alternative definition in Merriam-Webster describes anecdotal as "of, relating to, or being the depiction of a scene suggesting a story." With this definition, we see more clearly the value anecdotal evidence can offer to those who are astute and humble enough to listen.

In an article entitled "Value of Anecdotes" published in 2000 in the

Lancet, Rodger Charlton points out, "Publication in a scientific peer-viewed medical journal is unlikely to follow anecdotal observation. And yet in the *Lancet* of 1923 such observations were commonplace and at a time when major medical discoveries were being made." Anecdotes are not anathema to scientific progress. They are the starting point. They are scenes that suggest a story. At their heart, anecdotes are single observations in the physical world—and that is where science must always begin.

Returning to the anecdotal evidence I know best—my own—there is much information that can be mined from my experience with acne that you can use as a starting point to ascertain if fluoride is the source of your acne as well. First, let's talk demographics. I am a thirty-something adult and I am female. There is a common misperception that acne is a rite of passage for teenagers. This might have been the case a generation ago when fluoride was not as pervasive and older generations did not grow up with fluoridated teeth and bones. This is not the reality today.

Dermatologists and my hairdresser have both noticed the rise in adult acne, especially with women (Dreno 2015). In a 2012 study published in the *Journal of Women's Health,* researchers from Harvard Medical School recruited 2,895 females aged 10 to 70 from the general population and found that 55 percent had some form of acne, including 45 percent of women in their twenties, 26 percent of women in their thirties, and 12 percent of women in their forties (Perkins et al. 2012).

Acne can continue from adolescence or it can start in later years, a condition dermatologists refer to as late-onset acne. Dermatologists do not have an explanation for the observed increase in late-onset acne or for the rise in adult acne in general. However, this phenomenon is consistent with the fluoride theory of acne since it has long been recognized that fluoride accumulates in bone over time.* The more fluoride we consume, the more the rate of adult acne will increase.

---

*In parts of the world such as India and China where fluoride occurs naturally in drinking water, skeletal fluorosis is a common and debilitating condition and has been observed in areas where fluoride concentrations are equivalent to the current CDC recommendation for "optimally" fluoridated water (Dai et al. 2004; Connett 2012e).

The placement of your acne is another clue. I often developed acne in a line from the corners of my nose and mouth down to the bottom of my chin. Sometimes when dermatologists see this pattern they diagnose it as perioral dermatitis. *Peri* is from Greek and means "around." *Oral*, of course, means pertaining to the mouth. Dermatitis comes from *derma*, "skin," and *itis*, "inflammation." So when a dermatologist says you have perioral dermatitis, it's really just Greek caveman speak for "around mouth, skin bad, take drug."

Sometimes the lines of my acne breakouts extended from my nose all the way down the front of my neck, onto my chest. In a 2013 article entitled "Adult Female Acne: A New Paradigm," the authors note that in the rising tide of adult acne, "lesions are generally more prominent on the lower chin, jawline and neck" (Dreno et al. 2013). This pattern makes perfect sense since fluoride accumulates in the teeth and jaw, and then we brush, swish, and gargle with it twice a day. When my fluoroderma was at its worst, I also developed lines of acne from my ears down the sides of my neck, and from the base of my skull down the back of my neck. Sometimes I even developed clusters of acne on my forehead, and painful lumps around my ears and inside my earlobes.

A major clue in my self-diagnosis of fluoroderma was the realization that my breakouts were related to travel. Within two days of arriving at a new location, it was clear whether or not the new setting was going to be "one of those places." If your acne is conspicuously affected by travel, or if you notice a sudden onset or clearing of breakouts after moving to a new location, then that is an indicator your acne might be caused by fluoride. Once the idea of fluoroderma entered my mind, I was easily able to look back over my experience and see if my worst bouts of acne coincided with the cities where I was exposed to a higher level of fluoride. You can research whether or not towns are fluoridated by calling the local water municipality or looking up their annual water quality report online (also known as consumer confidence reports). Public water utilities are required by law to provide this information.

Another clue was my preexisting dental fluorosis. Remember the "grotesque brown stains" on the teeth of locals in the NIDCR's story of fluoridation? As the official story goes, "So severe could these permanent stains be, in fact, sometimes entire teeth were splotched the color of chocolate candy." (Leave it to dentists to come up with this analogy.) The extent of dental fluorosis seen today is rarely so severe, but any dentist will be able to recognize it. My dental fluorosis appears as bright white spots on the face of my teeth and an opaque quality around the edges. During my routine checkups, several dentists have also pointed out pitting and deep crevices, likely caused by the fluoride pills prescribed for me as a child.

Dental fluorosis only develops when fluoride is ingested in early childhood, when teeth are still being formed. When my permanent teeth came in, my parents asked my pediatrician about the discoloration, but he did not know the cause. I also developed chronic nosebleeds at this time, another indicator of fluoride toxicity. A survey released by the CDC in 2010 revealed 41 percent of adolescents aged 12 to 15 have dental fluorosis—that is roughly *twice* the rate they found in the same age group the decade prior (Beltrán, Barker, and Dye 2010). Dental authorities insist the condition is purely cosmetic. But as my favorite pagan dentist, Hardy Limeback, has stated, "It is illogical to assume that tooth enamel is the only tissue affected by low daily doses of fluoride ingestion" (2000).

None of the indicators above will prove or disprove that your acne is caused by fluoride. Not all adult females have fluoroderma and not everyone with fluoroderma is an adult female. Perhaps the location of my breakouts is specific to my particular history with fluoride and how it accumulated in my bones, teeth, and tissues. Maybe you don't have dental fluorosis, but you were exposed to high amounts of fluoride after your permanent teeth developed. Maybe your travels have not taken you to places where there was a significant difference in the amount of fluoride in the water supply, or maybe you consumed high amounts of fluoride that occurs naturally in some well water or from food sources.

That's the thing with anecdotal evidence. It requires further study to see how the observations drawn from one instance can be applied to others. You will need to figure out that part on your own. But because I *really, really, really* want to help you with it, I will tell you some other indicators of fluoroderma that are wrapped up in a dark secret I've scarcely whispered to a soul. They involve a side of acne that few people talk about, but even the experts have noticed.

LOST IN THE HUNDRED ACRE WOOD

I had breakouts throughout middle school and high school, but it wasn't until I went to college that my acne reached clinical proportions worthy of a visit to a dermatologist. For many of us, going away to college is the first time we move away from home. In situations like mine, it meant leaving a suburban or rural town for a more heavily fluoridated city center.

It can also mean roommates, housemates, exam stress, social stress, cafeteria food, fast food, no food, all-nighters, overnighters, new boyfriends, ex-boyfriends, and a thousand other factors that shape a new life away from home. In the midst of all this personal upheaval, it can be exceedingly difficult to make out the gorilla. But when I look back at my college experience, I see his footprints clearly, and they were on a decisively downward path. At the time, I had no choice but to follow him blindly. I now realize he was leading me on a pathway to depression.

College was the first time I distinctly remember having the feeling. It's not that I hated being there or even that I wanted to be anywhere else. It was just the first place I remember continually thinking, "What's the point?" The feeling tiptoed into my life sophomore year, but darted out of sight when I studied abroad in West Africa. After I returned to Georgetown senior year, it came into full view for the first time.

I remember my sweet college boyfriend sitting with me on a park bench in D.C., trying to explain how to feel happiness from watching birds take flight over the water. It sounded nice, but I just couldn't feel it. He bought me a small African violet plant that made me feel hopeful for some unidentified reason and a stuffed hippopotamus, which I admit I still cried into at night as a naval officer years later.

Crying at night was nothing new. In high school, I remember talking with a group of my girlfriends when one of them casually mentioned that she cried herself to sleep every night for absolutely no good reason. A bunch of us nodded our heads. Yep, that's normal. No cause for concern. We're girls. We cry. That's what we do. We all cry ourselves to sleep at night, and we all get acne.

If you visit the American Academy of Dermatology (AAD) webpage entitled "Tips for Managing Acne," like I did on February 16, 2017, you might notice something peculiar. The tips themselves are not surprising. Wash your skin twice a day. Keep your hands off your face. Don't pick. Don't scrub. Donate your money to dermatologists. Stay out of the sun. But after that, on the bottom of the page and without explanation, there is a link to a suicide hotline. When I clicked on it, it led to a stock GoDaddy page for a defunct website at suicidehotlines.com. But still.* Why is the AAD trying to send people reading about tips for clear skin to a suicide hotline? They don't do that for people searching for tips on how to deal with other major skin ailments. Why do they do it for acne?

The link between suicide and acne has long been documented in the medical literature. In a 1998 article published in the *British Journal of Dermatology,* researchers studied 480 patients with dermatological disorders and found those with mild to moderate acne experienced more suicidal thoughts than patients with atopic dermatitis, alopecia areata, or psoriasis covering up to 30 percent of their body (Gupta and Gupta 1998). The study excluded patients with cystic acne like mine, even though it is not uncommon. Other researchers report depression is two to three times more prevalent in acne patients than in the general population, and

---

*The link has since been fixed, but if you are struggling with thoughts of suicide, a more reliable resource is the National Suicide Prevention Lifeline available at www.Suicide PreventionLifeline.org or by calling 1-800-273-8255. (Hang in there, my friend. It might not feel like it now, but emotions are pliable. Keep turning the page. We'll figure it out.)

that women with acne, especially those over 36 years of age, experience depression over twice as often as men with acne (Uhlenhake, Yentzer, and Feldman 2010). In 2015, the British Skin Foundation released the results of their largest acne survey, revealing that out of 2,299 respondents, over 20 percent contemplated or attempted suicide.

The experts most often point to two contributing factors to explain the link between acne and depression. One of the factors is stress. In the title of a 2014 article published in the *Archives of Dermatological Research,* Rachel Albuquerque and her colleagues from the Federal University of São Paulo pose a promising question: "Could adult female acne be associated with modern life?" Their review notes the higher risks of depression among women and aims to establish a connection between the stress of the modern daily routine, sleep deprivation, and the recent increase in late-onset female acne.

It is true that college and the average work/life routine are stressful and that stress plays an undeniable role in health. On multiple occasions when I was particularly stressed over exams, I developed painful canker sores inside my mouth. (Could this be another indicator of fluoride toxicity?) But that only happened to me during exams at Georgetown or in the military. I never experienced stress-induced canker sores during graduate school in nonfluoridated Scotland.

The other common explanation for the link between depression and acne is low self-esteem. This one is so intuitive it is difficult to think past it. When you have ugly eruptions plainly visible on your face, it's only natural to feel self-conscious when interacting with other people. Few of us tend to react otherwise. In 1948, researchers published the first study examining the psychological impact of acne and concluded, "There is no single disease which causes more psychic trauma, more maladjustment between parents and children, more general insecurity and feelings of inferiority, and greater sums of psychic suffering than does acne vulgaris" (Sulzberger and Zaidens 1948). That is a powerful statement for a common skin condition known to come and go with time. There is one unproven word in their conclusion that completely changes our interpretation of what is going on with acne psycho-logically. If you reread their statement slowly you might notice it. (I will give you a hint—it's seven words in.)

The adage that "correlation does not imply causation" is a central con-cept in statistics and intelligence analysis alike. The principle is perhaps best illustrated in a spoof article on Bloomberg Business where the author depicts a graph correlating the rise of Facebook with the yield on ten-year government bonds in Greece (Chandrasekaran 2011). He also shows how the U.S. Housing Price Index mimics the increase in babies named Ava and how variations in the murder rate in New York state over time are a perfect match for the topography of an identified mountain range.

No matter how many studies show a connection between acne and stress, acne and depression, or even between acne and low self-esteem, these statistics cannot show *causality*. As with Cordain and his pseudo–*Star Wars* lexicon, medical researchers often give in to the temptation to dive into scientific literature and reverse–engineer a mechanism to show causality after a correlation has been established in the physical world. Their stories usually involve a lot of big words and microscopic characters that sound very convincing, but the rule stands. Correlation does not even *imply* causation. It is just as possible that acne, feelings of low self-esteem, and depression are all caused by an outside factor yet to be identified.

This is where your dual role as researcher and research subject really comes in handy. You don't need to interpret carefully worded questionnaires or quantify the varying levels of suicide-ness to deter-mine the details of your emotional state. You know your emotions in a way psychologists, psychiatrists, psychotherapists, dermatologists, den-tists, or any other -ists in existence ever could. You know the times you felt depressed—you were there. You know all the nuances of the dark thoughts that swim around your emotional states. You know the times you felt optimistic and carefree. And only *you* know the times you cried alone in a dark room wishing to fall asleep and not wake up.

My dark room was my bedroom in Newport, Rhode Island. There was so much going on in my life at the time, the idea that my depression was caused by my acne, let alone by low self-esteem from acne, never entered my mind. I was not happy about going into the military and felt manipulated into the predicament by my parents, who suggested I should at least take advantage of the first year of my full ROTC scholarship and then cancel without penalty if I decided the military was not right for me. Their proposal sounded reasonable, but they didn't mention that canceling the scholarship would mean dropping out of Georgetown, so I stayed even though military service did not appeal to me as a career.

The other major factor in my dark mood was the effect moving to Rhode Island had on my relationship with my college boyfriend—my first love and best friend—who was offered a dream job in New York City after graduation. We somehow held on in Newport and stayed together a couple years longer, but my tumultuous time in Rhode Island was the beginning of the downward trend of our relationship.

Wait a minute. What page is this? I feel like we might be too far into a science-y book without at least including a chart. Here is an exciting development! Since I originally wrote these lines, I found a publisher for my book who agreed to include a chart to illustrate this very point. The editors even insisted on using *two* charts so you can easily see how the high and low points correspond with each other. As the following charts show, the times of my life when I lived in a fluoridated area correlate with the times my acne was most severe. If you invert the chart, the high points correspond with the periods of my life I felt effortlessly happy, versus the times I felt overstressed from school, work, my personal life, or no identifiable reason at all.

The months I spent in Newport after graduation were my rock bottom. When I left, my mood steadily improved from "make it stop" back up to "what's the point" before hovering over "Melissa, just get through this" and finally reaching "maybe life will be okay after all someday far off in the future."

When I left the United States for Tunisia and Scotland, I started to feel good moods more regularly and without effort, unlike any time I could remember. I was sitting on a bench in St. Andrews when I very clearly realized that my life up to that point felt like a marathon, and I was exhausted from running it. I decided on that very bench that I was not going to let my life continue this way. I was going to stop running and start finding happiness in *this* moment. And I did. (If you haven't noticed this yet, declaring resolutions while sitting on benches bestows unexplained mystical powers—try it, you'll see.)

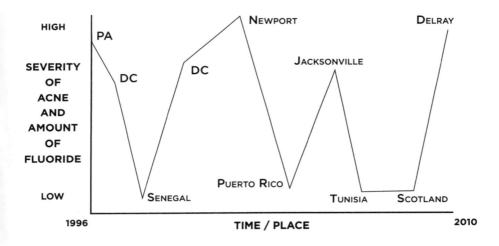

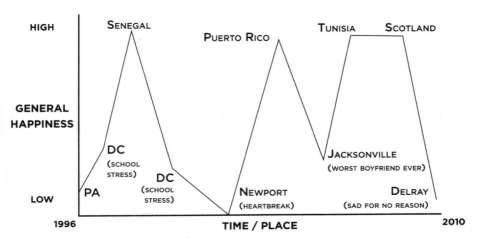

The times of my life when I lived in a fluoridated area correlate with the times my acne was most severe. If you invert the chart, the high points correspond with the periods of my life I felt effortlessly happy, versus the times I felt overstressed or depressed.

By the end of my time in Scotland, I had outgrown crying myself to sleep at night. I never cried at all anymore. Life was naturally exciting, and I was genuinely happy to be here. That is why I was shocked when I returned to the United States and my mood immediately plunged into murky but familiar waters. I had no reason to be apathetic about life. I was in love with my dream man who came as a package deal with my dream dog. I had just completed a Fulbright to the United Kingdom, an honor I never imagined I would achieve. And I was living rent-free in my favorite place on earth, the magical sunny kingdom of South Florida. I knew things weren't right when I lost interest in food. I still ate it, but it all seemed so boring and pointless. Rib eye, crab legs, summer berries. Blah. Normally I would feel at least a little sparkle of excitement with simple pleasures like these, but now everything just felt flat.

My boyfriend was the one who suggested maybe my acne was the cause of my depression. I didn't think so. Acne never bothered me like that before. All the other times I had acne I was depressed for *real* reasons. "You seem saddest on the days when your acne is the worst," he pointed out. It was true. Was I subconsciously so upset about my acne that it made me *lose all interest in life?* Could that happen without my approval? Doesn't the conscious me have a say?

I might have started to believe that acne was causing my depression if not for a few gorilla droppings left at the scene.

As I mentioned earlier, along with my graduate degree in International Security, I had officially started my master's in Health Nuttery while studying abroad in Scotland. By the time I moved back to Florida, I was doing a few things that we in the health nuttery field commonly refer to as "woo-woo health stuff," such as sleeping in total darkness in an attempt to regulate my hormones. The practice involved taking my oral temperature every morning before I got out of bed. It's normal for a woman's waking temperature to be lower before ovulation, but on some days it was remarkably lower than others, close to 97 degrees Fahrenheit. I noticed on days like this when my waking temperature was especially low, my mood was at its lowest point too.

This observation alone could have been written off as a coincidence, but there was another sign that told me something systemic was going on with my depression. Multiple times after having a really low day, I noticed white marks on my fingernails a day or two later. I've had similar white spots on my nails off and on my whole life, but these were so pronounced and the timing so suspicious that I decided to ask my good friend Internet about them.

I came across a Q&A from Andrew Weil (2005), a popular Harvard-trained medical doctor who walks the line between conventional and alternative approaches to health. A reader asked him if the spots are indicative of a mineral deficiency. Weil pulls a common medical doctor tactic by first demonstrating his expertise on the subject (you've probably seen this one before) by busting out some fancy Greek caveman talk to explain that white spots on fingernails are referred to in the medical field as leukonychia, which according to my trusty Greek caveman dictionary (it's Google) translates back into English as the name of the legendary punk metal band, "White Nail."

Weil goes on to explain that the marks are usually caused by us crazy knuckleheads knocking our hands on random junk and forgetting about it, or maybe it was a rough manicure or a reaction to nail polish (you know, girl stuff). He closes his expert advice by dispelling some rumors that are making the rounds amongst us kids these days. It is a myth that leukonychia is caused by calcium deficiency, zinc deficiency, or Hellman's mayonnaise. "I'm not making this up," he attests. He sounds serious about that last part, so I believe him.

But the rest of his explanation about the origins of white marks on fingernails did not resonate with my experience of them. Why did I get pronounced white spots on my nails when my mood flatlined and my face broke out? Why didn't I get them in Scotland? Why do some people get white marks on their nails and others do not? I wondered why Weil was so confident in his assessment of the causes of leukonychia. I wondered why doctors are confident in their assessment of anything—how do they know what they *think* they know?

I couldn't envision Weil ever taking the time or effort to test his theories on fingernails in the real world. His explanation seemed like a mashup of the one I read on Wikipedia and one written seven months before Weil's article by a mystery commenter who debunked the Hellman's mayo myth and was posted in an online forum (pinky swear be damned) at SalonGeek, "the world's largest community of salon professionals dedicated to open discussion, personal development, and powerful passion for the industry we love" (Geek 2004).

The white marks on my fingernails reminded me of something. I went to my thinking spot to think, think, think. Ah, I remembered. When I took fluoride pills as a child while my teeth were forming, it showed up as bright white spots on my tooth enamel. Could the same thing be happening with my fingernails? I asked Internet about "fluoride and leukonychia," but she was uncharacteristically quiet on the topic—prolly thought I was showing off.

Then I asked her about "fluoride and fingernails," and she offered a 1999 study by researchers at the Medical College of Georgia who measured fingernail clippings to see if they can be used as a biomarker for subchronic exposure to fluoride (Whitford, Sampaio, et al. 1999). They found that a month of increased fluoride intake resulted in significant increases in fluoride concentrations of fingernail clippings after a lag time of approximately 3.5 months. I was on to something. I asked Internet, "Real quick, how long does it take for fingernails to grow from nail bed to tip." She answered via Wikipedia: 3 months, at least.

The white marks on my nails, my low waking temperature, my acne, my depression, and my consumption of fluoride were all correlated. There was evidence that fluoride could be *causing* the white marks on my nails, and I was already vetting the idea it was causing my acne. I formed a testable hypothesis: if fluoride was the cause of my low waking temperature and my depression, then limiting fluoride in my diet should increase my waking temperature and get rid of my depression. The white marks on my fingernails, along with my acne, should disappear for good too.

I steadily tested my hypothesis over the next few years, and that is exactly what happened. Now that I know how to limit my fluoride exposure, I don't have acne, I don't have white marks on my fingernails, and I don't have depression. Am I just knocking my hands around less and not using them to pick at my bacteria-laden face? Is my life that much better than it was a few years ago that it's now effortless to be happy?

Life is still stressful. I still work long hours, I have an arduous commute and a lot of work-related travel, there's drama with my family, and I'm putting all my free time into writing this book. But clear skin comes naturally for me now and so does happiness. Here's my secret: that is how it should be when you're *not being poisoned*.

CHAPTER 42*

Now this is where our story really gets exciting; we have cause for a *second* chart. And not just any chart. We need the mother of all science charts. The periodic table of the elements.

Looking at the periodic table on page 68, you will see the F for fluorine at the top of the second to last column on the right. It sits at the head of a group of elements called halogens. The halogen group consists of fluorine, chlorine, bromine, iodine, and astatine. The name halogen means "salt-producing" and was given to this group because of their tendency to react with metals to produce a wide range of salts, including calcium fluoride (a mineral that spawned the word fluorescence), sodium chloride (common table salt), and potassium iodide (what they add to salt to make it "iodized").

To the right of the halogens is a group of elements called the noble gases. This group consists of helium, neon, argon, krypton, xenon, and radon and was given the name noble gases because they do not like to mingle with others. They used to be called inert gases, but scientists later observed that on very rare occasions noble gases can bond with other elements, mostly fluorine because of its extremely high reactivity.

---

*If you ask Internet, "What is the answer to life?" she will tell you it is 42. Go ahead. Try it and see. (FYI, this is foreshadowing for chapter 6.)

1	2	3	4	5	6	7	8	9	10	11	12	13	14	15	16	17	18
1 **H** Hydrogen 1.008																	2 **He** Helium 4.003
3 **Li** Lithium 6.94	4 **Be** Beryllium 9.012											5 **B** Boron 10.81	6 **C** Carbon 12.011	7 **N** Nitrogen 14.007	8 **O** Oxygen 15.999	9 **F** Fluorine 18.998	10 **Ne** Neon 20.180
11 **Na** Sodium 22.990	12 **Mg** Magnesium 24.305											13 **Al** Aluminum 26.982	14 **Si** Silicon 28.085	15 **P** Phosphorus 30.974	16 **S** Sulfur 32.06	17 **Cl** Chlorine 35.45	18 **Ar** Argon 39.948
19 **K** Potassium 39.098	20 **Ca** Calcium 40.078	21 **Sc** Scandium 44.956	22 **Ti** Titanium 47.867	23 **V** Vanadium 50.942	24 **Cr** Chromium 51.996	25 **Mn** Manganese 54.938	26 **Fe** Iron 55.845	27 **Co** Cobalt 58.933	28 **Ni** Nickel 58.693	29 **Cu** Copper 63.546	30 **Zn** Zinc 65.38	31 **Ga** Gallium 69.723	32 **Ge** Germanium 72.630	33 **As** Arsenic 74.922	34 **Se** Selenium 78.97	35 **Br** Bromine 79.904	36 **Kr** Krypton 83.798
37 **Rb** Rubidium 85.468	38 **Sr** Strontium 87.62	39 **Y** Yttrium 88.906	40 **Zr** Zirconium 91.224	41 **Nb** Niobium 92.906	42 **Mo** Molybdenum 95.95	43 **Tc** Technetium [97]	44 **Ru** Ruthenium 101.07	45 **Rh** Rhodium 102.906	46 **Pd** Palladium 106.42	47 **Ag** Silver 107.868	48 **Cd** Cadmium 112.414	49 **In** Indium 114.818	50 **Sn** Tin 118.710	51 **Sb** Antimony 121.760	52 **Te** Tellurium 127.60	53 **I** Iodine 126.904	54 **Xe** Xenon 131.293
55 **Cs** Cesium 132.905	56 **Ba** Barium 137.327	* 57 - 70	71 **Lu** Lutetium 174.967	72 **Hf** Hafnium 178.49	73 **Ta** Tantalum 180.948	74 **W** Tungsten 183.84	75 **Re** Rhenium 186.207	76 **Os** Osmium 190.23	77 **Ir** Iridium 192.217	78 **Pt** Platinum 195.084	79 **Au** Gold 196.997	80 **Hg** Mercury 200.592	81 **Tl** Thallium 204.38	82 **Pb** Lead 207.2	83 **Bi** Bismuth 208.980	84 **Po** Polonium [209]	85 **At** Astatine [210]	86 **Rn** Radon [222]
87 **Fr** Francium [223]	88 **Ra** Radium [226]	** 89 - 102	103 **Lr** Lawrencium [262]	104 **Rf** Rutherfordium [267]	105 **Db** Dubnium [270]	106 **Sg** Seaborgium [269]	107 **Bh** Bohrium [270]	108 **Hs** Hassium [270]	109 **Mt** Meitnerium [278]	110 **Ds** Darmstadtium [281]	111 **Rg** Roentgenium [281]	112 **Cn** Copernicium [285]	113 **Nh** Nihonium [286]	114 **Fl** Flerovium [289]	115 **Mc** Moscovium [289]	116 **Lv** Livermorium [293]	117 **Ts** Tennessine [293]	118 **Og** Oganesson [294]

	57 **La** Lanthanum 138.905	58 **Ce** Cerium 140.116	59 **Pr** Praseodymium 140.908	60 **Nd** Neodymium 144.242	61 **Pm** Promethium [145]	62 **Sm** Samarium 150.36	63 **Eu** Europium 151.964	64 **Gd** Gadolinium 157.25	65 **Tb** Terbium 158.925	66 **Dy** Dysprosium 162.500	67 **Ho** Holmium 164.930	68 **Er** Erbium 167.259	69 **Tm** Thulium 168.934	70 **Yb** Ytterbium 173.045
*Lanthanide series														
**Actinide series	89 **Ac** Actinium [227]	90 **Th** Thorium 232.038	91 **Pa** Protactinium 231.036	92 **U** Uranium 238.029	93 **Np** Neptunium [237]	94 **Pu** Plutonium [244]	95 **Am** Americium [243]	96 **Cm** Curium [247]	97 **Bk** Berkelium [247]	98 **Cf** Californium [251]	99 **Es** Einsteinium [252]	100 **Fm** Fermium [257]	101 **Md** Mendelevium [258]	102 **No** Nobelium [259]

Fluoride is a highly reactive, unstable element in the halogen group.

About a century ago, serious scientists like chemists and physicists realized the number of electrons in the outer shell was a governing factor in how elements bond with each other and their level of reactivity. The reason for the unusual chemical stability of the noble gases is because, with the exception of helium, they each have a full octet of electrons in their outer shell. Scientists concluded that all elements are continually trying to reach the stable state that comes with having eight electrons in their outer shell, as epitomized by the noble gases.

The entire periodic table is set up around this principle, with elements in each column forming groups that reflect the number of electrons in their outer shells. Group 1, headed by hydrogen (H) located all the way on the left, only has one electron in their outer shell. This lonely electron is easily lost, explaining why elements in this group are so unstable and why you should always fill your blimps with helium, a noble gas, instead of hydrogen, from whence the term H-bomb is derived.

Continuing along our periodic table from left to right, elements in each column increase their outer electron count by one. So Group 2, headed by beryllium (Be), has two outer electrons. The "transition metals" in Groups 3 to 12 get weird with this, so scientists try to tuck them all in together and then, acting as if nothing strange happened, continue along with Group 13, the boron (B) group, which has three electrons in their outer shell, and so on. If you keep counting, you'll see that Group 17, the halogens, has an outer shell with seven electrons—so close to nobility! Fluorine, more than any of the other halogens, wants to be king *so bad* he'll do whatever it takes. All he needs is one more lousy electron in his outer shell and the kingdom is his. (Pause here for dramatic effect.) This missing electron is what makes fluorine so unstable.

Fluorine is more reactive than other halogens because it is the lightest. Elements at the top of their group in the periodic table have the smallest atomic weight, a property that increases as you descend down each column. This is why people make the claim that fluoride is the most reactive element on the planet.

Chemists nicknamed fluorine "the tiger of chemistry" because it kills so many overconfident chemists in the lab. Dentists, on the other hand, like to point out that fluoride is a naturally occurring natural mineral, that it exists naturally in virtually all natural water supplies, and that Nature herself chose it as the thirteenth most abundant natural element in the Earth's natural crust, naturally. But now you know there is more to the story. Fluoride's abundance explains why it is the by-product of so many big industries, and its high reactivity explains why it causes so many damaging health effects throughout the human body.

Government bodies like the U.S. Public Health Service (PHS) have been caught passing notes in class with statements like "Fluoride: An Essential Mineral Nutrient" (1974). Contrary to PHS rumors, nutrients are commonly defined as biochemical substances that provide energy or building material for the survival and growth of a living organism. A nutrient is considered essential if it must be obtained from external sources. This is not the case with fluoride.

When essential nutrients are restricted from the diet, predictable side effects develop. For example, if you can't sleep at night, your skin turns pale and mysteriously starts blistering at the thought of sunshine, blood drips from your swollen mouth, and you become aggressive to the point of insanity, you might need to beef up on your B3 intake (Hampl and Hampl 1997). Unlike with B vitamins, there is no evidence that restricting fluoride in the diet has any negative effects on the body whatsoever, even on teeth, therefore it is not considered an essential nutrient.

In fact, there is little evidence that fluoride is even a nutrient. As you will learn in the next chapter, there are a lot of foods in the modern diet that contain significant amounts of fluoride, but in the majority of cases—tea leaves being the prime exception—the fluoride found in our food supply is not naturally occurring. Most of it comes from pesticides and from the pollution of phosphate fertilizer plants that dental devotees insist we all use to drink, bathe, and wash our underwear (so creepy).

Even fluoride that occurs naturally in some water sources is more a matter of geology than biology. If the water happens to run through fluoride-heavy rocks such as cryolite or bauxite, then it too will contain high amounts of fluoride. This is why deep water wells are more likely to contain significant doses of fluoride than most spring water sources. People in certain parts of India, China, and elsewhere suffer severe health consequences because of naturally occurring fluoride in their water supply (Connett 2012e).

Mother Nature gave us a big clue about the place of fluoride in the human diet when she installed what one study in the *British Medical Journal* describes as "a physiological plasma-milk barrier" that prevents fluoride from being passed to breastfeeding infants (Ekstrand, Boreus, and de Chateau 1981). If fluoride is helpful for growing strong teeth, why does Mother Nature withhold it from us at the time we would need it most? Knowing her, that doesn't sound like something she would do.

While there is no evidence that indicates fluoride is an essential nutrient, another member of the halogen group, iodine, clearly is. Individuals with severe iodine deficiency develop an enlarged thyroid gland visible as a swollen protrusion around their neck, a condition known as goiter. In severe cases, a lack of iodine can result in cretinism, a condition characterized by the lack of both physical and mental development.

A less recognizable sign of iodine deficiency is hypothyroidism, a common disorder of the endocrine system where the thyroid gland does not produce enough thyroid hormone. Symptoms of hypothyroidism include dry skin, cold hands, *low body temperature,* fatigue, irritability, mental haziness, constipation, and weight gain. It is worth noting that women with melasma, the dark facial pigment I developed when using benzoyl peroxide for my acne, are found to be four times more likely to have hypothyroidism (Lute et al. 1985). The experts disagree on how many people in the United States have underactive thyroid glands, but they do agree the number is well into the millions and that the majority are women. Harvard researchers predict one in five women will develop hypothyroidism by age sixty (Harvard Health Publishing 2011).

Iodine and fluorine are located at opposite ends of the halogen group. Since iodine is the heaviest of the halogens found in the human body (and the heaviest of all elements needed by living organisms), it loses out to other halogens that compete for the same receptors. When we have high amounts of fluoride in our diets, especially when iodine is lacking, our bodies absorb fluoride where they would normally absorb iodine. For example, until the 1950s, doctors in Europe and South America prescribed fluoride to *reduce* thyroid activity in patients with *hyper*thyroidism (Galletti and Joyet 1958). They found that a dose as low as 2 to 5 milligrams per day over a period of a few months decreased thyroid activity in their patients.

Fluoride's propensity to displace iodine explains why fluoride causes such a wide variety of negative health effects. Discussions of dietary iodine tend to focus on the thyroid gland, but iodine is needed throughout the glandular system, including in the breasts, ovaries (which also produce thyroid hormone), pancreas, thymus, salivary glands, and so forth. Fluoride competes with iodine for receptors in these glands, as well. In the late 1990s, Jennifer Luke, a doctoral candidate in the United Kingdom, dissected eleven human pineal glands and discovered that calcified portions of the gland contain the highest concentrations of fluoride in the human body—up to 21,000 ppm (Luke 1997). The pineal gland secretes melatonin and helps regulate the seasonal and circadian rhythms of the body.

As with acne, there is a documented link between hypothyroidism and depression. A 2006 study published in the *American Journal of Psychiatry* examined 142 adult patients with major depressive disorder who did not achieve remission even after two optimally delivered trials of antidepressant medications (Nierenberg et al. 2006). The study found that 25 percent of test patients who received a thyroid hormone supplement went into remission for their depression after just 14 weeks. The clear role of iodine and the thyroid gland in mental health could at least partially explain the correlation between acne (aka fluoroderma) and depression. It also sheds light on the mysterious role played by hormones in the development of acne. Dermatologists, teenagers, and women with eyes and brains have noticed a correlation between acne and hormonal fluctuations caused by puberty, menstruation, birth control pills, and pregnancy. The official explanation doesn't go much beyond the idea that certain hormones make your face shiny,* but there must be more to the story than that.

The human body does not restrict its use of iodine to the endocrine system. Concentrations of iodine are also found in cerebrospinal fluid and throughout the brain (Adrasi et al. 2003). When Phyllis Mullenix, the prominent toxicologist and fluoridation pagan discussed in the previous chapter, began studying fluoride, the existing scientific literature led her to believe fluoride, unlike iodine, does not cross the blood-brain barrier. But she was suspicious of previous studies because they administered fluoride via injection and then measured fluoride content of the brain an hour later (Mullenix 2000). To more accurately reflect

---

*According to information presented at the American Academy of Dermatology's 70th Annual Meeting by Bethanee Schlosser, director of Women's Skin Health at Northwestern University, the key hormonal factor in understanding acne is as follows: "Androgens, the male hormones present in both men and women, can contribute to acne flares by overstimulating the oil glands and altering the development of skin cells that line hair follicles in the skin." (As cited at AAD.org, "Hormonal factors key to understanding acne in women," March 16, 2012.)

the way humans are chronically exposed to fluoride in the water supply, she conducted an experiment by giving 532 rats fluoridated water and then measuring the fluoride content of their brains several *weeks* later (Mullenix et al. 1995).*

Mullenix and her team were shocked when they discovered major accumulations of fluoride in every section of the brain. Their studies show that rats with postnatal exposure to fluoride exhibit symptoms of *hypo*activity while those with prenatal exposure to fluoride exhibit symptoms of *hyper*activity. This evidence prompted the growing concern that fluoride could be a contributing factor in the prevalence of Attention Deficit Hyperactivity Disorder (ADHD) in the United States, a claim supported by recent demographic studies comparing rates of ADHD and fluoridation (Malin and Till 2015).

In a 2012 meta-analysis of the scientific literature on the neurotoxicity of fluoride, Harvard researchers reviewed twenty-seven studies on the subject and found that all but one showed a significant link between higher levels of fluoride in the water supply and reduced IQ (Choi et al 2012). As Caroline Martinez, a pediatrician and researcher at Mt. Sinai Hospital in New York, explains, "Fluoride appears to fit in with a pattern of other trace elements such as lead, methylmercury, arsenic, cadmium, and manganese—adverse effects of these have been documented over time at exposures previously thought to be 'low' and 'safe'" (as quoted in Main 2015b).

These are just a few of the adverse health effects caused by fluoride exposure. The full list is much more extensive because every cell, organ, and tissue in the human body evolved using iodine—an abundant element in ocean water—in place of fluoride, which modern industry

---

*You might be surprised when you see that the rats in Mullenix's study received water containing fluoride at 100 ppm. This confused the dentists too. Because of her training in toxicology, Mullenix knew to begin her studies by using animal doses that produce a level of fluoride in the plasma equivalent to that found in humans drinking fluoridated water and using fluoridated dental treatments. Her efforts to conduct follow-up studies were not funded, and she was dismissed from her position when her research brought into question the safety of fluoridation.

has unearthed in unnatural proportions from deep within the Earth's crust. I have not even touched on fluoride's role in arthritis, rheumatoid arthritis, bone fractures, certain types of cancer, infertility, kidney disease, fibromyalgia, and many other debilitating conditions that plague our industrialized society.* Even though you are likely reading this book because you want to heal your acne, acne is not the root problem. Like these other disorders, it is a symptom of chronic fluoride poisoning—a term I don't use for dramatic effect, but because it is appropriate.

When you look at your acne as a symptom of a larger story, you will have a better vantage point for observing the full picture of how fluoride is affecting your body. When my fluoroderma was at its worst, acne was not the only physical sign something was very wrong. In addition to depression, I often had a thick oily residue in my hair. When I went for acupuncture, the doctor remarked on the whiteness of my tongue and called in her assistant to show her. In traditional Chinese medicine, a thick white coating on the tongue represents excess dampness in the body. In addition, my breath smelled bad even though I brushed and flossed more and made an extra effort to stay well hydrated.

Since I'm putting it all out there at this point, I might as well tell you I had bad body odor too. When I lived acne-free in Senegal, I forgot to pack my special hypoallergenic deodorant, so I went without it for nearly a year in one of the hottest countries on earth. I might have been sweaty, but I never remember smelling bad, and my roommate swore I didn't either. In Delray Beach where the water was heavily fluoridated, I smelled bad sitting in the air conditioning all day.

Speaking of hypoallergenic deodorant, skin sensitivities are another potential indicator of fluoride toxicity. The reason I couldn't simply purchase a new deodorant when I forgot mine is because in high school I developed severe skin sensitivity to most deodorants. I also had skin reactions to laundry detergents, fabric softeners, shaving cream, body

---

*For more information about fluoride's role in various health conditions, visit http://fluoridealert.org/issues/health

scrubs, the little moisturizing strips on razors, and probably a bunch of other chemical products I was never able to identify. These are the kinds of little quirks you might not bother mentioning to doctors and if you did they would have no idea what to tell you. But whether the clues provided by your health conditions are big or small, they help tell the story of your body in a way only *you* might ever be likely to decipher.

For example, when I moved to Jacksonville, Florida, I developed a recurring rash on my right forearm. It came and went many times, but I couldn't figure out the cause. I asked a military doctor about it at a routine physical. He in turn asked if I used one of those poof things in the shower. I said I did, and he told me I was probably scrubbing too hard. I didn't say anything at the time, but something in his answer made me wonder how closely he was paying attention during his poof class at medical school. My incessant intelligence analyst brain wondered why the rash only appeared on my right arm. Wouldn't I naturally scrub harder on my left arm since I am right-handed? And why didn't the rash appear elsewhere I scrubbed with my left arm since I was likely scrubbing those areas with the same intensity? (See how annoying intelligence analyst brains can be?) I left Jacksonville for nearly a year, during which time the rash never came back, but when I returned to Jacksonville it quickly made a reappearance.

Now that I know more about how the human body responds to fluoride and my particular history with it, I can easily develop my own hypothesis about the mystery rash on my arm. Perhaps the location of the rash is because I broke my right forearm when I was in kindergarten and the bone bioaccumulated additional fluoride during the healing process since that was the same time frame when I was ingesting fluoride pills. Perhaps the timing of the rash is because I purchased a cheap mattress in Jacksonville from a mattress discount warehouse that I suspect sprayed their piles of unwrapped mattresses (it was seriously discounted) with either fluoride-based pesticides or bromine-based flame retardants or both. Bromine is another dangerous halogen we'll discuss in an upcoming chapter.

I didn't figure out the mattress connection until it went into storage for a couple of years and then ended up in a guest room in my current house. When we were painting our master bedroom, my husband and I slept in the guest room, and after a two-year absence, the mystery rash again made a reappearance. It was the first time I ever saw it outside of Jacksonville, so I knew the cause was something I brought with me. A doctor would never have been able to put all these clues together, but because they involve small details of my everyday life, I am naturally the expert in such matters.

And so are you.

HAPPILY EVER AFTER

There are a lot of blank pages we still need to fill before we reach the end of our story. An important part of any analysis is trying to identify and articulate your known intelligence gaps. With regard to my analysis of fluoroderma, one intel gap is that I don't know what percentage of acne in the general population is caused by fluoride. But I suspect it is a significant portion.

When George Waldbott, the renowned allergist and early fluoridation pagan, published his series of case reports and double-blind studies in the 1950s, he found that 1 percent of the population experienced hypersensitivity to ingested fluoride from the water supply. His findings were replicated by the largest government-funded clinical trial of fluoride supplements, which confirmed that 1 percent of children given a daily 1 milligram fluoride tablet—the amount contained in one liter of water fluoridated at the recommended level—exhibited adverse reactions such as eczema, atopic dermatitis, and hives (Feltman 1956).*

---

*You might be wondering why the government funded a critical study of fluoridation, but there is a completely logical explanation. They didn't realize that is what they were doing. The U.S. Public Health Service ceased funding for the study prior to its ten-year target date because they thought it was supposed to be a study "to determine the efficacy (in preventing caries) of the addition of measured doses of fluoride salts to pregnant

If 1 percent of the population in 1950s America was hypersensitive to fluoride, in the absence of contemporary follow-up studies, we can only extrapolate what that statistic might be today. We have endured seventy years of public water fluoridation, fluoride-based pesticides are pervasive in the food supply, and we live with fluoridated teeth and bones inherited from our parents not through genetics but through the cultural inheritance of a government health system that failed to outsmart industry influence and then got caught up in its own fiction. We have been living with fluoridation for so long, it has literally become a part of who we are. None of us know what our skin—or our society— would look like without it.

In the 1990s, a cunning but unwitting group of Finnish dentists provided a rare glimpse of how the cessation of public water fluoridation would affect the rate of skin conditions in the general population. The town of Kuopio, Finland, with 83,000 inhabitants, was the only town in the Nordic countries to fluoridate its water supply. After thirty-three years of antifluoridation campaigning that climaxed in bitter local disputes, the city council finally agreed to discontinue fluoridation in 1992. Dentists at Kuopio University Hospital sensed an opportunity to expose the alleged health complaints associated with fluoride as psychological manifestations of an ignorant populace. They devised a plan to discontinue fluoridation early without informing the public and then to study the occurrence of various symptoms among a group of people who believed that the piped water was still fluoridated even though it was not.

There was little chance the Finnish dentists would see the gorilla in his tutu who was about to dance across the stage.* In their study published in a 1997 issue of *Community Dentistry and Oral Epidemiology*,

---

(cont.) women and children." They were not interested in funding studies on the adverse health effects of fluoride. The study continued anyway and the results were published in the *Journal of Dental Medicine* in 1961 after fourteen years of investigation (Feltman and Kosel 1961 as quoted in Connett 2010).

*First author to ever write that line. . . . I called it.

the authors point out their own preconceived bias: "The results obtained were mostly expected and, in our opinion, quite convincing . . . it seems likely that the prevalence of the symptoms considered in the current study is connected with the psychological rather than with the physical effects of being exposed to fluoridated water" (Lamberg, Hausen, and Vartiainen 1997). Oh, dentists. Why do you make us do this to you? Let's take a closer look at this one last study before we move on to the next part of our story.

In November, when people in Kuopio knew the water was still fluoridated, the dentists sent one thousand surveys asking for recipients to check a box next to a list of twenty-five symptoms to indicate those they were currently experiencing (acne was not one of the choices). In December, they sent another thousand surveys to a separate group of people who were unaware that the amount of fluoride in the water had returned to natural levels three weeks prior. In March, they sent the same survey again to both groups. All recipients were between the ages of 25 and 64, excluding two of the most susceptible demographics. (That's fine. Whatever. Moving on.)

When comparing the differences in the rates of reported symptoms between November when the first group knew the water was fluoridated and December when the second group only thought it was fluoridated, the difference was found to be *highly significant* for one symptom: "other skin rash." Did the dentists focus on this information in the summary of their findings? No, that was not the story they expected—or wanted—to tell. But between pontifications on the psychological antics of antifluoridationists, the dentists admit, "The significant decrease in the number of other skin rashes leaves room for speculation [author note: telling word choice there, no?], seeming to favor the view that a small segment of the population may have some kind of intolerance to fluoride. This group of people should be studied further [but not by us obviously]." FYI, I added that last part for emphasis.

Furthermore, the entire Kuopio study is based on the dentists' stated assumption that symptoms of chronic fluoride poisoning will pass as quickly as symptoms of acute fluoride poisoning. I'm not a toxicologist (or a dentist who pretends to be a toxicologist), so I am relying on my little layman brain here, but I would not assume the symptoms of thirty plus years of chronic fluoride poisoning would be completely alleviated after three weeks. Aren't the mechanisms for acute poisoning and chronic poisoning different?

For example, if a child suffers acute fluoride poisoning after accidentally swallowing a fraction of an ounce of bubblegum-flavored toothpaste, she would likely experience symptoms of the flu such as stomach pain, headaches, nausea, and vomiting that would clear in a few days at most (Connett 2012a). In contrast, a woman in India who is about to develop severe skeletal fluorosis from chronic fluoride poisoning due to fluoride in her water supply would exhibit symptoms of joint pain and stiffness similar to arthritis ("Skeletal Fluorosis in India and Its Relevance to the West" 2012). No one would expect the symptoms of the prefluorosis woman in India to clear after just three weeks or even three months of receiving nonfluoridated water.

My most severe fluoroderma flare-ups lasted up to a month, and it took me a few years to figure out how to clear my acne completely. The questions on the Finnish survey were all yes or no. Either you had depression and joint pain from one month to the next, or you did not; there was no room for anything in between.

If you will indulge my analytic tendencies a bit further, it would be insightful to take a moment to make an assessment of our assessments on the health studies we have examined in more detail thus far. You might have noticed a common theme running through our conclusions. In the chocolate bar study, the paleo studies with the Kitavan/Ache/Melbourne participants, the Grand Rapids experiment, and now this Finnish survey, the researchers from all of these efforts got into trouble when they stopped reporting on *what* they were observing and started reporting on *why*. It wasn't the natural world that was steering them wrong, it was their interpretation of it.

Researchers are human (even dentists) and as such are limited by the cognitive traps we all face. My ulterior motivation for looking at these studies with you so closely is to demonstrate that it doesn't take a degree in medicine to put forward a thoughtful assessment of the researchers' conclusions. Scientific literature can look overwhelming with all the sacred words, charts, and statistics, but there is usually enough English for anyone reading this book to follow along with whatever story the authors of scientific studies are telling. With Internet's help, we have the opportunity to add our previously muffled voices to the dominant conversation on acne and health in general. That is why I've tried to include links to every study I referenced—to encourage you to go to the source and look at the evidence yourself with your unique vantage point, fresh eyes, and your little layman brain.

Another intelligence gap is that we do not know if there are other dietary elements that cause acne, and if so, how those elements affect the development of fluoroderma. Even if I were the only person in the world who experiences acne from ingested fluoride, my case study would still evidence the fact that acne, at least in certain situations, is caused by diet—a reality most dermatologists refuse to accept. As hard as it is for dermatologists to believe, the existence of even just one case of fluoroderma shows there must be a physical mechanism in place for certain substances that enter your body through your mouth on their way to your stomach to be broken down into smaller components and then somehow circulated to other areas of your body, sometimes ending up all the way back up around your mouth where they started. (Some researchers speculate the existence of such mechanisms and refer to them simply as the digestive and circulatory systems.)

We do not know if other elements use these same mechanisms to cause acne. In *The Hidden Plague,* our fellow health investigator, Tara Grant (2013), describes how she discovered that nightshades, a family of flowering plants that includes tomatoes, potatoes, eggplant, and peppers, among others, were the cause of her acnelike skin condition known as hidradenitis suppurativa. Nightshades contain chemical compounds called alkaloids, which evolved as natural pesticides to protect the plants from bugs and predators. Similar to fluoride, some of the strongest evidence of nightshade sensitivity is its connection to arthritis and joint pain (Childers and Margoles 1993). Could it also be a hidden cause of acne? And what is its relation, if any, to fluoride intoxication?

Other signs indicate a connection between acne and additional foods that commonly cause food sensitivities, such as grains, gluten, sugar, soy, and dairy (I have a hypothesis for that last one; will explain soon). The absence of certain elements can cause skin problems, as well. For example, the lack of iodine has a clear effect on skin health, as does zinc deficiency. An imbalance of bacteria in the digestive system might also play a role. Our analysis of Cordain's hormonal theory of acne shows how some of these connections can be confused with fluoroderma. Once fluoride is removed from the equation, it will be easier for researchers—including you—to assess any other potential acne culprits.

Which brings us to the most important intelligence gap in our analysis: we do not know the source of *your* acne. I am confident in my assessment that fluoride was the cause of mine, but I do not know if it is causing yours. Our time together has been brief thus far, and you've patiently allowed me to monopolize our whole conversation. You now know all the details of my travel history, my secret depression, even the spots on my fingernails—but I know very little about you. And yet your part in the story of acne is *the most important*. Your experience will help determine if fluoride-induced acne is an anomaly or if my assessment is accurate that acne is a condition of Western civilization because of our chronic fluoride intoxication. The ending of our story can only be written by you.

The best way to diagnose fluoroderma is through direct observation of fluoride's effect on your skin. Some people ask me about blood or urine tests to gauge fluoride sensitivity. While those tests do exist, you don't need a test to tell you how your skin reacts to fluoride. You can just look in the mirror. Fluoride tests are not common in the United States, and the results would leave a lot of room for interpretation as to their ramifications for your acne. For example, if you measured the amount of fluoride in your urine, it would only show a minuscule picture of what is going on with fluoride in your body. It will not tell you if you have fluoroderma or high amounts of fluoride in your teeth, bones, plasma, or other tissues.

It is not a coincidence that the most effective test for fluoroderma is also the simplest. Like the PHS researchers who tested for fluoride sensitivity by giving children 1 milligram of fluoride per day and then observing its effect, once you know the common sources of fluoride in our industrialized life, you can readily observe how your skin reacts after you are exposed to them. Since most people in America are already overwhelmed by fluoride exposure, the safest way to gauge your sensitivity is to start eliminating major sources of fluoride and see if your skin improves. Initially, it is important to look for a reduction in acne rather than a complete elimination, as it is difficult to root out hidden sources of fluoride all at once.

An easy way to begin is to stop using fluoridated toothpaste and mouthwash. Nonfluoridated versions are available at any health store. If your fluoroderma is triggered purely by topical contact, then your acne will completely heal with this one simple move. Although dentists and dermatologists rarely mention this, there is a body of scientific literature documenting the causal relationship between topical applications of fluoride and perioral dermatitis (Connett 2012d), a condition that was never reported until the mid-1950s during the early years of fluoridation (Mellette, Aeling, and Nuss 1983).

To address the deep cystic welts, you will need to lower the amount of fluoride you are consuming in your diet. You could begin by reducing your consumption of artificially fluoridated drinking water. In part 2, we will discuss how to determine if your water source is fluoridated and if so, what options are available to reduce your exposure.

If you have masochistic tendencies, you could confirm your fluoroderma in one step by eating a low-quality chicken hot dog or wonton soup prepared from a cheap chicken carcass, although I do not recommend it. These were the sources of my most severe fluoroderma flare-ups and resulted in cystic breakouts a few hours later around my jaw and down the front, back, and sides of my neck. As with humans, chickens are not immune to the bioaccumulation of fluoride from their pesticide-laden food supply.

There is one last intelligence gap I would like to point out. For the most part, throughout my assessment of fluoroderma thus far I've tried to focus on the tangible evidence that shows fluoride is the root cause of acne while refraining from theoretical explanations of *why* fluoride causes acne. As we've seen in our examinations of previous health studies, the *why* can be a much more complicated question to untangle. We know fluoride is a highly reactive element and that it bioaccumulates in various parts of the human body following exposure in unnatural proportions, including in teeth and bones. We know fluoride and iodine are both halogens and that they both have an effect on hormones, particularly thyroid hormones. We also know iodine is essential for healthy skin and mental well-being. But why does long-term fluoride ingestion lead to skin eruptions? What exactly is going on inside our bodies that causes fluoride to end up on our faces? I have a theory but I'll save it for a little later.

What I do know is that the *whats* and the *whys* dermatologists have been professing since the advent of dermatology are not a full or even an accurate depiction of the story. Dermatologists still claim that a proximate cause of acne is that we have excess oil on our skin because our oil glands are overproductive. These are such relative terms, *excess* and *over*productive. Maybe our bodies have good reason to produce extra oil upon certain hormonal cues. Maybe our glands are perfectly productive under the current circumstances.

Dermatologists describe acne as a disease, but what is a disease *really?* My experience with fluoroderma leads me to believe that acne is not a disease. Our oil glands and our hormones—and our bodies—are not malfunctioning. They are functioning exactly as they should be, given their environment and the raw material provided. You are not in a fight against acne; you're on the same team. If not for acne, I would not have healed my depression by learning how to avoid fluoride. Each breakout was a signpost pointing the way back to physical and emotional health.

Acne is not a disease to be treated. It is a message to be heard. Our role is to stop and listen.

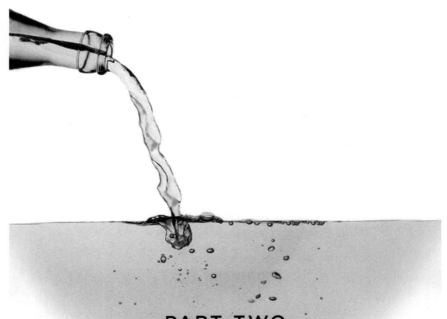

PART TWO

~~~~~

Affect (*v.*)

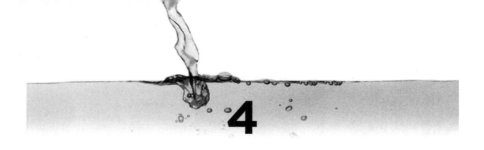

4

Stopping Breakouts
Before They Start

"But I don't want to go among mad people," Alice remarked.
"Oh, you can't help that," said the Cat: "we're all mad here.
*   I'm mad. You're mad."*
"How do you know I'm mad?" said Alice.
"You must be," said the Cat, "or you wouldn't have come
*   here."*

LEWIS CARROLL,
ALICE'S ADVENTURES IN WONDERLAND

IF YOU ARE INCLINED TO TRUST health authorities, it can be unpleasant to realize the CDC is an unwitting Queen of Hearts shouting "off with their heads" while living in a house of cards.

It can be even more disconcerting to learn the cystic welts on your face are caused by common tap water. The everyday world takes on new shades of danger. You start to wonder about the free glass of ice water at a restaurant. Maybe you notice an unsettling feeling as you sink into a warm bath. The double ristretto venti decaf caramel frappuccino from your favorite coffee shop is eyed with new suspicion.* Once you suspect fluoride is causing your acne, the world around you doesn't look the same. But it won't always be that way.

---

*Does Starbucks contain fluoride? To find out, see www.HiddenCauseofAcne.com/does
-Starbucks-contain-fluoride

Preventing acne should be as effortless for you as it is for a Kitavan. The long-term solution is to end artificial water fluoridation and demand more responsible use of fluoride-based pesticides (see appendix: The Plan). But you don't have time right now to move your pawn-self across the whole chessboard for a chance to rewrite the royal decrees. You need to start healing your acne *today*.

Artificial water fluoridation will end—and I predict it will be our generation that makes it happen—but you don't have to wait until then before you can live acne-free. Once you understand where fluoride comes from and how it makes its way into the industrialized food supply, you will know how to choose foods and drinks that are naturally low in fluoride. You will know, for example, that beer and wine can both contain significant amounts of fluoride but for different reasons. More importantly, understanding those reasons elucidates how to choose options that will not contribute to future breakouts.

When I was lying on my couch in Delray Beach with my raw face painted in yogurt, I wished for a computer printout of every factor that was causing my acne. I thought it was an impossible dream at the time,[*] but three years later I realized I was printing its fulfillment when I made a hard copy of an online cheat sheet I created to help other people suffering from fluoroderma.[†]

Dentists use the fact that fluoride is found throughout the food supply to demonstrate its safety, but you will soon see the weakness in that argument. At first glance, the list of fluoride sources appears to be a random assortment of foods, drinks, and other arbitrary means of fluoride exposure. But things aren't always as they seem. There is a logic behind the madness, and it is readily deciphered by curious minds.

---

[*]No, I do mean impassible. Nothing's impossible.
[†]To receive a copy of the cheat sheet, visit www.HiddenCauseofAcne.com/guides

THE DRINK ME POTIONS

Let's begin at the beginning with fluoridated water and then, as the Red King decrees, we will go until we come to the end and stop.

As I mentioned in part 1, fluoride in water can occur naturally, or it can be added artificially at local water treatment plants. Well water will absorb fluoride naturally if it runs through fluoride-based rock. Since fluoride is the thirteenth most abundant element in the Earth's crust, naturally fluoridated water is not an uncommon occurrence. A known fluoride belt stretches from Syria through Jordan, Egypt, Libya, Algeria, Sudan, and Kenya. Another extends from Turkey through Iraq, Iran, Afghanistan, India, northern Thailand, and China.

Deep water wells and those at the foot of high mountains are particularly susceptible to fluoride accumulation, but individual wells throughout the United States and elsewhere have also been found to contain high amounts of fluoride. A 2008 report from the U.S. Geological Survey notes that 4 percent of sampled wells in the United States exceed the EPA's secondary maximum contaminant level for fluoride of 2 ppm (DeSimone, Hamilton, and Gilliom 2009).

The CDC recommends having your well water tested for fluoride at least once every three years and urges alternative drinking water sources if the level of fluoride is greater than 2 ppm (2015). Your skin, however, will likely disagree with that number. An amount under 0.1 ppm is more desirable. A survey conducted by Canadian environmental officials found the average fluoride content of fresh surface water such as lakes, rivers, and springs to be 0.05 ppm (Health Canada 1993). The average fluoride content of rainwater is even lower at 0.008 ppm (Mahadevan, Meenaksy, and Mishra 1986).

If your residence is connected to a public water municipality, you can confirm the fluoride content by researching the most recent water quality report, also known as consumer confidence reports. All community water systems are required to provide a full water quality report to their consumers every year. You can often find them online or by calling your local water utility.

The Environmental Protection Agency has a website to assist with finding your consumer confidence reports online, but sometimes it's easier to make a phone call.* Speaking with your water provider directly can offer additional insight you might not find in the official report. For example, you could ask them where they purchase the fluoride they add to the water supply and what type of fluoride is used. When my mom called her water supplier in Pennsylvania, she was told they temporarily stopped adding fluoride because of a shortage. When I called Seacoast Utility Authority while visiting Palm Beach Gardens, the receptionist told me the local community (one of the wealthiest neighborhoods in South Florida) is ardent that fluoride not be added to the water supply.

Many water treatment personnel are well educated on fluoride and are personally and professionally against fluoridation. It is only natural to be suspicious when you see for yourself the skull and crossbones on the containers. Water workers are the ones required to physically handle the chemicals, whether they agree with the practice or not.

If your water is fluoridated, you have two near-term options for refusing force-fed fluoridation. One option is to drink bottled water verified to be low in fluoride. This was the course I pursued when I first suspected fluoride could be the cause of my acne. As with local water utilities, you can determine the fluoride content of various bottled water brands by researching their water quality reports online, or you can contact the manufacturer directly. They should have this information readily available. Per FDA labeling requirements, if bottled water is labeled as deionized, purified, demineralized, or distilled, it will only contain fluoride in trace amounts unless fluoride is specifically listed as an added ingredient.[†]

Besides bottled water, the other option is to invest in a filter that

---

*For help finding your local water quality report, visit www.HiddenCauseofAcne.com /resources

†See "Bottled Water and Fluoridation" available at www.cdc.gov/fluoridation/faqs /bottled_water.htm

removes fluoride from your regular water supply. Common carbon filters like Brita and Pur do not reduce fluoride, but reverse osmosis systems, deionizers, activated alumina, and distillation will remove most if not all fluoride from your drinking water. For more information on filters to remove fluoride, see www.HiddenCauseofAcne.com/fluoride-filters.

Fluoridated water is just the beginning, unfortunately. Now our story gets twistier. To simplify matters, here is a mnemonic device to help remember the five primary drinkable sources of fluoride exposure. You can count them on one hand as some of the most memorable characters from *Alice in Wonderland*. Our sordid cast of fluoridated potions includes Tweedledumb,* Tweedledee, the Red Queen, the White Rabbit, and of course, Johnny Depp (a.k.a. the Mad Hatter).

If fluoridated water is Tweedledumb, then beverages made with fluoridated water are his equally contrariwise twin brother, Tweedledee. Soft drinks, juice, iced tea, coffee, and other beverages can all be made with fluoridated water, and if so they will contain fluoride in amounts equal to or higher than the water with which they were produced.

Researchers at the University of Iowa measured fluoride concentrations of 332 soft drinks and found over 70 percent contained fluoride at levels exceeding 0.6 ppm (Heilman et al. 1999). Researchers in New Zealand examined 532 juices and juice drinks and found fluoride levels ranging from .02 to 2.8 ppm (Kiritsy et al. 1996). The researchers in both studies accounted for the wide range of fluoride in large part because of variations in the amount of fluoride of the water used in production, proving Tweedledee right all along when he said, "If it was so, it might be; and if it were so, it would be; but as it isn't, it ain't. That's logic."

Beer falls in the Tweedledee category. If it is made from fluoridated water, it will contain fluoride. In 2002, researchers at King's College in London measured the fluoride content of various brands of beer, lager, and cider available in the United Kingdom (Warnakulasuriya et al. 2002). They found a range of fluoride from .06 to .71 ppm and

---

*Yep, the *b* is intentional.

concluded that alcoholic beverages can be a significant source of fluoride even though they were not accounted for in the Total Diet Study when British officials estimated the average daily fluoride intake of its citizenry at 1.82 ppm (Walters et al. 1982). The British officials who conducted the fluoride portion of the Total Diet Study—two of whom hailed from the Ministry of Agriculture, two of whom hailed from the Laboratory of the Government Chemist, and one of whom was named Sherlock—did not suspect alcoholic beverages as a source of total dietary fluoride intake among British citizens and yet diligently accounted for fluoride in the tail meat of krill. Curiouser and curiouser, is it not?

If you don't have time to research the fluoride content of beer in advance, those brewed in continental Europe are generally a safe option since 97 percent of western Europe does not fluoridate its water supply.

Following Dumb and Dee is the Red Queen: wine. According to measurements from the 2005 USDA National Fluoride Database of Selected Beverages and Foods, wine contains an average fluoride content of 1.05 ppm for red wine and 2.02 ppm for white wine (USDA 2005). But these numbers tell us very little about the amount of fluoride contained in the bottle of wine on your kitchen counter. To understand that, it helps to know where the fluoride in wine comes from. Whereas beer is made from brewing certain grains in water, wine is made from crushing grapes. There's no water added.

The reason wine can contain significant amounts of fluoride is because of another Wonderlandesque character, the Western Grapeleaf Skeletonizer. A caterpillar exactly 3 inches tall with conspicuous tufts of long black poisonous spines, they feed on the undersides of grape leaves before transforming into luminescent blue-winged fairies.* The Omnivorous Leafroller, a bell-shaped character with a gray batlike snout and brown ombre wings, is also to blame. To limit crop damage from Western Grapeleaf Skeletonizers and Omnivorous Leafrollers,

---

*Or moths, whatever. The University of California claims Western Grapeleaf Skeletonizers are only 0.6 inches in length, but I defer to Lewis Carroll in all matters of caterpillar measurement.

some grape growers use a pesticide called cryolite, which acts as a deadly poison in their grapeleaf-greedy bellies.

Cryolite was already featured in our story, just not by name. In the official version of the story of fluoridation outlined in chapter 2, the young dentist hero's interest in fluoride was sparked when he realized it was the cause of the townspeople's brown teeth, a condition known as "Colorado Brown Stain." In Colorado Springs, where our hero settled, the community watershed was high in fluoride because it contained deposits of cryolite from the rock formations of Pike's Peak. This is the same mineral, sodium hexafluoroaluminate, that is crushed and sold to grape growers under the trade name Kryocide, although now it is widely produced synthetically by combining sodium, fluoride, and aluminum.

Here's where your newfound insectology knowledge is put to good use. You see, Western Grapeleaf Skeletonizers and Omnivorous Leafrollers tend to confine their grape-leaf dining activities to California's Central Valley. To outsmart the Red Queen at her own game, all you need to do is choose wines from vineyards outside this region.

According to the California Department of Pesticide Regulation's online database, the use of cryolite on wine grapes is generally confined to four counties in southern San Joaquin Valley: Fresno, Kings, Tulare, and Kern. Northern vineyards, including those in Napa and Sonoma, do not use cryolite. Neither do vineyards in southern or coastal areas like Temecula or Monterey.

To confirm, I wrote to every regional winery and growers association in California outside San Joaquin Valley and asked about their use of cryolite. Those who replied either had never heard of cryolite or verified they do not use it. I was also told that since cryolite is a fluoride product, some agricultural chemical companies like Wilbur Ellis won't sell it because of possible problems with residual fluoride in the ground-water.* On neighboring chessboards in Oregon and Washington states,

---

*October 19, 2015, email message to author from Josie Gay, Executive Director, Heart of Sonoma Valley Winery Association.

vineyards are not treated with cryolite either (see "No Worries About Cryolite Here" 2007).

My skin verifies this information. I can drink wine from Sonoma, Columbia Valley, Europe, Argentina, New Zealand, and elsewhere without incident, but when I tried to politely sip a glass of California wine when visiting at a friend's home, my skin broke out before I left her house. Years later, I learned why. The winery is located in San Joaquin Valley.

In 1989, valiant challengers from abroad threatened the Red Queen's reign by limiting the fluoride content of all wine exported to Europe to 1 ppm. In response, Elf Atochem North America, the manufacturer of Kryocide, joined with other dark knights (i.e., Gowan Company, Gallo Winery, the Wine Institute, and California State University–Fresno) to joust for an exception for California vineyards that use cryolite by raising their limit to 3 ppm—an amount that is 50 percent higher than the Maximum Secondary Contaminant Level set by the EPA and over four times higher than the CDC's current recommendation for fluoridated water. Their efforts were successful, and yet some California vineyards treated with cryolite still fail to meet the 3 ppm exception (see "Kryocide Advisory on Use of Cryolite to Control Insects on Grapes" n.d.).

The Red Queen monarchy extends to grape juice made from this region, as well. In a study of forty-three ready-to-drink fruit juices, researchers from Tufts University measured the highest amount of fluoride in grape juice from the baby food company Gerber at 6.8 ppm, well above the EPA's already inflated maximum contaminant level for fluoridated water of 4 ppm (Stannard et al. 1991). Even fruit juices and other fruit drinks that don't have the word *grape* in their name often contain blends of grape juice that include significant amounts of fluoride.

In 2002, a cryolite supplier petitioned the National Organic Standards Board to have it included on the list of allowed pesticides for organic production (Formella 2002). You can tell the petition was proofread by dentists because of phrases like "as a mineral, the only residues remaining are basic elements found in nature," and also because of the A+ cartoon tooth sticker at the top of the page. Despite this strong argument, the petition was rejected and as a result, organic fruit juices contain the least amount of fluoride, since the use of cryolite is prohibited on organic crops.*

But don't forget about Tweedledee and his propensity to confuse matters. If juice is made with fluoridated water it can still contain fluoride even if it is labeled as organic. "If it was so, it might be." Got it?

The next character in our lineup is the White Rabbit. If you follow him deep enough down the rabbit hole, he will eventually reveal the whole matrix. He first hops across the page when Alice chases him into Wonderland, the same way researchers chase dairy down the rabbit hole of dietary causes for acne.

In 2005, a study headed by a nutritional epidemiologist from Harvard School of Public Health analyzed questionnaires from 47,355 teenage females from the famous Nurses' Health Study and found a positive correlation between acne and dairy consumption, particularly skim milk (Adebamowo et al. 2005). His team published follow-up studies in 2006 and 2008, both of which supported the correlation between milk consumption—especially skim milk—and adolescent acne.

Dermatologists were confused by these results. If milk causes acne in adolescents, surely it must have something to do with the hormones milk contains. In his response to the Harvard study published in the same journal issue, dermatologist Guy *"Sassypants"* Webster begins, "Diet causes acne. [*snap*] No it does not!"† He then argues that the study's findings "seem to exonerate bovine hormones as the acne factor in milk because they would presumably be mostly in the lipid fractions" (2008). In other words, whole milk should cause more acne than skim milk because of its higher fat content, and thus its higher hormone content; therefore, diet is not the cause of acne; therefore, drugs are the only solution. But that does not appear to be what is happening in the wonderland of acne research.

---

*For information on the history of substances, including cryolite, petitioned for inclusion on the National Organic Standards list, see the USDA website at http://www.ams .usda.gov/rules-regulations/organic/national-list/co
†Sass in italics added for emphasis.

To understand what is going on with milk and acne, it helps to ponder a question posed to Alice at a certain tea party you might remember her attending, uninvited. "Why is a raven like a writing desk?" Excellent question, don't you think? It leads one to wonder what makes one thing, one thing and another thing, the other thing save someone says it's so. Why is milk, milk and not a raven or a writing desk?

If you ask the U.S. Food and Drug Administration, the answer is very clear. According to the U.S. Code of Federal Regulations Title 21, Section 131.110, milk is "the lacteal secretion, practically free from colostrum, obtained by the complete milking of one or more healthy cows."* It is unclear what the resulting liquid is called following an incomplete milking of a goat who is feeling a little under the weather, for example, but their definition sounds reasonable enough so far.

The guidelines go on to explain that milk "shall contain not less than 8¼ percent milk solids not fat and not less than 3¼ percent milkfat." That seems unnecessarily demanding of both God and Mother Nature, but okay. They continue, "Milk may have been adjusted by separating part of the milkfat therefrom, or by adding thereto cream, concentrated milk, dry whole milk, skim milk, concentrated skim milk, or nonfat dry milk." In Section 133, Subpart A, under the definition of milk used for cheese, they add, "Water, in a sufficient quantity to reconstitute concentrated and dry forms, may be added."†

To quote the headline of a 2000 article by Emily Green in the *Los Angeles Times*, "Is milk still milk?" If you ask Wikipedia, your grandmother, a suckling baby, or even the FDA-equivalent in another country, the definition of milk you receive will likely be a little different, and probably a lot simpler. According to Wikipedia, "Milk is a white liquid produced by the mammary glands of mammals." The end. As you can see, the FDA definition stretches this concept of milk much further.

---

*21 CFR 131.110 can be found at http://www.gpo.gov/fdsys/pkg/CFR-1999-title21 -vol2/pdf/CFR-1999-title21-vol2-sec131-3.pdf
†21 CFR 133.3 can be found at http://www.gpo.gov/fdsys/pkg/CFR-1999-title21-vol2 /pdf/CFR-1999-title21-vol2-sec133-3.pdf

Virtually all words—*milk, raven, writing desk, bac'n bits*—are brimming with this kind of existential wiggle room that shrewd food manufacturers use to their advantage. What if the teenagers in the Harvard study weren't drinking milk at all, like that guy in *The Matrix* who sold out Neo for a digital steak? What if they only *thought* they were drinking milk, but it was really an imposter made of the same stuff as chocolate-chip-*flavored* cookies or powdered country *lemonade*.*

Humpty Dumpty elucidates this point quite eloquently when he tells Alice, "When I use a word, it means just what I choose it to mean—no more, no less . . . I can manage the whole lot of them! Impenetrability!"

In her article for the *Los Angeles Times,* Emily Green (2000) describes the Frankenstein process industrialized milk goes through to be recreated after leaving the udder. First, it is shipped to a processing plant where centrifuges are used to separate it into fat, protein, and various other solids and liquids. Once segregated, they are then reconstituted to standardized levels for whole, low-fat, and skim milks. "Whole" milk is the closest to original cow's milk, but it's still not the same thing, and it's certainly not whole. When skim milk is first produced it is a watery, chalky, blue-tinged shadow of real milk's natural self, which is why some people still refer to it as "Blue John." As one traditional dairy farmer put it, the product in the grocery store we commonly think of as milk is no longer milk, but rather it is a reconstituted milk-flavored beverage.

According to the USDA National Fluoride Database of Selected Beverages and Foods (2005), skim milk has a mean fluoride concentration of 0.03 ppm. The same is true for milk with 1 or 2 percent milkfat. But mean averages don't mean much in Wonderland where there are only four branches of Arithmetic: Ambition, Distraction, Uglification, and Derision. As the Red Queen has already demonstrated, government measurements of the fluoride content of various

---

*For more fake foods, see "19 Foods that Aren't Foods" by Mandy Oaklander, *Prevention,* July 1, 2013, at http://www.prevention.com/food/19-foods-arent-food

foods are meant to be more of a nonsensical guideline than a respectable gauge of the amount of fluoride contained in the product you just purchased at the grocery store.

To make skim milk palatable and more acceptable aesthetically, manufacturers add powdered milk solids. Could powdered milk solids—not hormones—be the reason industrialized skim milk-flavored beverages are correlated with acne? Researchers tend to go on and on about dairy as if ravens and writing desks have *so much* in common, but the studies on powdered milk solids are scant, and studies on the fluoride content of powdered milk solids are even scanter. Let's see if we can find some clues.

In the original Harvard study, other dairy products found to have a positive correlation with acne were cottage cheese, cream cheese, instant breakfast drinks, and sherbet. Each of these products is commonly made from skim milk or contains milk protein concentrates. (You don't even want to know what kind of dairy goes into what the FDA classifies as sherbet.)* In the USDA fluoride database, milk solids are not listed, but powdered cream substitute is noted as having a mean fluoride concentration of 1.12 ppm. In a 1952 article entitled "A Survey of the Literature of Dental Caries," the authors reference a study conducted ten years prior

---

*Fine, don't listen to me. Here it is: "(b) Optional dairy ingredients. The optional dairy ingredients referred to in paragraph (a) of this section are: Cream, dried cream, plastic cream (sometimes known as concentrated milkfat), butter, butter oil, milk, concentrated milk, evaporated milk, superheated condensed milk, sweetened condensed milk, dried milk, skim milk, concentrated skim milk, evaporated skim milk, condensed skim milk, sweetened condensed skim milk, sweetened condensed part-skim milk, nonfat dry milk, sweet cream buttermilk, condensed sweet cream buttermilk, dried sweet cream buttermilk, skim milk that has been concentrated and from which part of the lactose has been removed by crystallization, and whey and those modified whey products (e.g., reduced lactose whey, reduced minerals whey, and whey protein concentrate) that have been determined by FDA to be generally recognized as safe (GRAS) for use in this type of food. Water may be added, or water may be evaporated from the mix. The sweet cream buttermilk and the concentrated sweet cream buttermilk or dried sweet cream buttermilk, when adjusted with water to a total solids content of 8.5 percent, has a titratable acidity of not more than 0.17 percent calculated as lactic acid. The term 'milk' as used in this section means cow's milk." Source: 21 CFR 135.140 (Frozen Desserts).

(before fluoridation) when researchers found the fluorine content of cow milk solids to vary from 0.4 to 4.4 ppm (Jeans 1953).

So how much fluoride is commonly contained in milk solids? I'm not sure anyone knows. In a 2012 study published in the *British Journal of Nutrition,* researchers in Iran found high levels of fluoride in certain powdered milk formulas and concluded they were likely caused by water used in the factory during the production process (Mahvi 2012). Skim milk solids are widely manufactured through a technique called spray drying. In this technique, the milk is processed as a slurry in a rotating cylinder before being dehydrated. The Iranian researchers postulate that when the water from the slurry vaporizes, fluoride remains concentrated in the finished product. If their theory is correct, milk solids processed in plants with fluoridated water would contain higher amounts of fluoride than other milk solids.

We are deep in the rabbit hole now, and I can't say with certainty if we will reach the other side. It is possible dairy products correlate with acne for reasons other than the fluoride content of milk solids, or perhaps they do not correlate at all. My skin cannot attest to the fluoride content of industrialized milk products because I have not consumed them since discovering my fluoroderma.* I still drink milk and eat plenty of cottage cheese, yogurt, and other dairy products daily, but they are not the morphed variety found only in Wonderland.

Instead of purchasing milklike beverages at the grocery store, the majority of my dairy products are now delivered fresh from a traditional farm (i.e., where cows live on pastures), just like when my grandfather was a milkman in the 1940s and 1950s before the industrial needs of World War II fully reshaped the American diet—and before acne was an accepted part of everyday life. If you decide it is time to wake up from Wonderland altogether, you can learn more about how to locate a dairy farmer near you by visiting www.HiddenCauseofAcne.com/food-supply.

---

*You might be wondering why I don't just drink some skim milk and see what happens— you know, in the name of science. Truth is, I made the mistake of reading *Skinny Bitch* several years ago, and now I can never drink grocery store milk again.

The final character in our drinkable lineup is the colorful, lovable, mad-as-a-hatter Hatter. After failing to impress the Queen of Hearts with his rendition of "Twinkle, Twinkle, Little Bat," the Hatter is sentenced to death for "murdering the time." He escapes, but time is unforgiving and halts the Hatter at six o'clock in the evening, leaving him in a perpetual tea party, a Victorian version of Margaritaville.

Studying the topic of fluoride and tea is enough to drive one mad. Remember that statistic dentists like to quote about how fluoride is the thirteenth most abundant natural element in the Earth's crust? Tea plants happen to be the only edible plants that uptake natural fluoride from the soil in large amounts, so of course that's the one we decide to build our empires around.* The amount of fluoride in a single cup of tea varies widely. Most studies report levels from 1 to 5 ppm depending on the age of the plant, the chemical characteristics of the growing region, and the length of steeping time (Ruan and Wong 2001).

In 2010, researchers from the Medical College of Georgia discovered the fluoride content of tea is even higher than previously thought. Four patients were each diagnosed with skeletal fluorosis because of their advanced joint pain and excessive tea consumption (FYI, one will only be diagnosed with skeletal fluorosis if one's symptoms are advanced and one's fluoride consumption excessive).† When researchers measured the amount of fluoride in the brands of tea the patients were drinking, however, they were puzzled to find the concentrations were very low. Where was the fluoride that was causing their skeletal fluorosis?

Realizing that tea also absorbs inordinate amounts of aluminum, the researchers wondered if the aluminum was somehow hiding the fluoride. They performed an experiment to test their hypothesis by dissolving the insoluble aluminum fluoride bonds found in tea prior to measuring for fluoride. Their results showed that fluoride concentrations in seven

---

*Sarah Rose, *For All the Tea in China: How England Stole the World's Favorite Drink and Changed History* (New York: Penguin Books, 2011).
†For more information, see fluoridealert.org/studies/tea03

common store-bought brands of black tea were up to three times higher than previous measurements indicated.

To be clear, the type of tea we are discussing here is tea from the *Camellia sinensis* plant. It commonly comes in black, green, and white varieties with white being the lowest in fluoride since the leaves are picked when young. Ceylon, pekoe, oolong, pu-erh, Darjeeling, Earl Grey, instant—these are all ways of referring to tea from the *Camellia sinensis* plant and thus are susceptible to fluoride accumulation.

Some sources claim organic tea is lower in fluoride, but I have not found any information to confirm that assertion. High-quality matcha tea from Japan is said to be low in fluoride, as well. In theory tea plants grown without soil (i.e., hydroponically) could be cultivated to have low levels of fluoride, but I do not know of any that are commercially available.* Truthfully, I have not looked very hard because I already switched to herbal tea by the time I realized my acne was caused by fluoride.

Herbal tea is another raven/writing desk situation. Technically, it's an infusion, or tisane, which is defined simply as a drink prepared by soaking the leaves of a plant in liquid. This description would seem to apply to tea as well, but tea experts assure us it does not. Tea is tea and tisanes are not tea. If enough of us nod in unison then it will be declared so, as is the case with all language. Tea that is not tea includes peppermint, chamomile, dandelion, and many other flavorful varieties. I find the taste of raspberry leaf is a nice substitute if you are craving traditional black tea. If you drink tea for an energy boost, my sensei, Tim Ferris, recommends yerba maté.

So there you have it. The five common drinkable sources of suspected fluoride exposure are fluoridated water (Tweedledumb), beverages made with fluoridated water (Tweedledee), wine from the Fresno

---

*In a 2013 article by Chinese researchers studying the fluoride content of hydroponically grown tea plants, they found the aroma of the tea leaves decreased as the fluoride content increased, leading them to conclude that "elevated concentrations of [fluoride] during growth have negative effects on the aroma and flavor quality of tea leaves" (Li et al. 2013).

region of California (the Red Queen), frankenmilk (the White Rabbit), and tea (the Mad Hatter). But before we move on to the next scene, there is more we can learn about fluoride from the experience of hatters.

Prior to the mid-1900s, hatters were a mainstay of society for centuries. Someone had to create all the fashionable hats everyone thought they were required to wear while out in public. Hats were made from the pelts of small animals which the hatters turned into felt by removing the fur from the skin. Respectable hat manufacturers claimed to use camel urine to break down the necessary chemical bonds in the pelts. Unfortunately for hatters and hat wearers, camels aren't the thirstiest of creatures and sometimes camel urine was hard to come by in places like France and England. When faced with camel urine shortages, resourceful hatters used their own instead (Kitzmiller n.d.).

Over time, French hatters made a curious observation. If a hatter happened to have syphilis and happened to be taking mercury chloride as a treatment for the disease, his urine was especially effective at making felt. How fortuitous.

Hatters started using mercury, a known neurotoxin, for felting, and soon afterwards phrases like "mad as a hatter" came into common usage. Symptoms of mercurial poisoning were prevalent amongst hatters and included insomnia, depression, loose teeth, digestive problems, shaking so severe it inhibited basic functions like walking and speaking, paranoia, mental instability, miscarriage, hallucination, and early death (Clark 1997).

In 1860, a physician in New Jersey named J. Addison Freeman published an article entitled "Mercurial Disease Among Hatters" that outlined the illness and recommended steps for prevention, which were promptly ignored by the American hatmaking industry and government regulators (Freeman 1860 as quoted on Wikipedia). In 1878, an inspection of twenty-five hat companies in Newark found that a quarter of the 1,589 hatters exhibited mercurial disease (Dennis 1878). By the turn of the century, both France and Great Britain passed legislation to protect hatters from mercury poisoning, making the condition rare in those countries, but American hatters continued going mad for decades.

By 1934, the U.S. Public Health Service estimated that 80 percent of American felt workers, most of whom were poor immigrants, suffered from mercurial tremors. Yet the practice did not end until *nine years later* when hat manufacturers volunteered to use hydrogen peroxide, a readily available substitute, since mercury supplies were needed to produce detonators for World War II (Wedeen 1989).

There are a number of lessons from our mad-hatter history we can apply to our current experience with fluoride. First, just because an expert at the top of his profession thinks something is a good idea, it does not mean it is safe for humans. He might turn out to be a crazy French hatter with syphilis (or a dentist).

Second, as with fluoride, mercury is a natural element that occurs naturally in the Earth's natural crust, ranking just behind silver in natural abundance. Clearly, just because an element is natural does not mean it is safe for humans.

Third, it took the United States government over eighty years after the publication of Freeman's article on mercurial disease among hatters (plus a *little* extra incentive from WWII) to end the use of mercury in the hatmaking industry, showing that just because a practice has been in widespread use for decades *does not mean it is safe for humans*. When we decide to do something dumb, sometimes we keep on doing it for a very long time. (You know this.)

Finally, in his account of mad-hatter syndrome in New Jersey, Richard Wedeen notes the most remarkable aspect of the hatters' story is that they expressed no anger about their working conditions. The minutes from their association meetings make no reference to any of the symptoms of mercurial poisoning. The medical community, the government, the general public, and the hatters themselves all seemed thoroughly unconcerned by the raging lunacy exhibited by the people creating their pretty hats. So is the case with fluoride.

As the wise Cheshire Cat explained to young Alice, everyone is mad in Wonderland. It's to be expected.

Tweedledumb and Tweedledee
Fetch only plain tap water.
Fresno's Queen, White Rabbit scheme,
Mad Hatter's tea is hotter.

THE EAT ME CAKES

I have to admit, the *Alice in Wonderland* theme seemed like a fun and fitting analogy, but now that I'm digging into it, I'm starting to wonder something. All the references to fluoride are starting to seem a little more than coincidental, you know what I mean?

Take Alice's encounter with Humpty Dumpty, for example. She meets him sitting there on top of the wall and you know exactly where that chapter is going. None of the king's horses or even his men could put Humpty back together. If you repeat the words of the nursery rhyme and then close your eyes and picture Humpty Dumpty, what do you see? An egg? Wrong! Humpty Dumpty was a cannon. It was used in Colchester, England, in 1648 during the English Civil War until an opposing cannon knocked down the wall beneath it, causing Humpty to fall to the ground, never to be recovered (Wears 2014). Go ahead and repeat the nursery rhyme again. See? No egg.* Lewis Carroll is the one who is credited with turning Humpty Dumpty into a story about broken eggshells. And guess what's high in fluoride. Yep. Eggshells.

As with humans, birds bioaccumulate fluoride. In an article published in the *Journal of Wildlife Diseases,* researchers in Norway measured fluoride concentrations in 405 herring gull eggs and discovered that eggs found near aluminum smelters were significantly higher in fluoride. They also measured for fluoride in forty-two herring gull femur bones and found a positive correlation between the amount of fluoride

---

*"Humpty Dumpty sat on a wall. Humpty Dumpty had a great fall. All the king's horses and all the king's men couldn't put Humpty together again." See? Still no egg. But it does leave one wondering why they named their cannon Humpty.

in a bird's femur bone and in the shells the bird produced (Vikoren and Stuve 1996). Researchers in Poland performed similar tests on domestic hens. The bones from chickens who drank fluoridated water were significantly higher in fluoride than the bones of chickens in a control group (Machaliński 1996).

Why should you care if the chickens you eat are bioaccumulating fluoride? Most people don't eat eggshells or chicken bones, right? Wrong again! (What's up with you today?) Most people do eat chicken bones, they just don't know it, and they are consuming outrageous amounts of fluoride at the same time.

Chicken caused my absolute worst acne flare-ups. Soon after diagnosing my fluoroderma, my husband and I decided to move to a neighboring county that is nonfluoridated. I was excited about simple things like being able to take baths again and order soup at a restaurant. While we were still house hunting, I made the mistake of ordering wonton soup from a local Chinese takeout place. Within hours, my face was Freddy Krueger. I called the water company who verified the water was nonfluoridated, and then I called the restaurant to ask about the soup. They proudly explained it was made in the traditional manner by simmering a chicken carcass for several hours to make a mineral-rich broth. Ah-ha! That explained it. I was basically eating dissolved chicken bones.

I had a similar experience after accidentally purchasing chicken hot dogs instead of the regular beef version I usually bought. It was a high-quality brand made from "all-natural" chicken raised without antibiotics or artificial hormones, but none of that mattered.

Chicken hot dogs and other chicken products are often made from an industrialized product referred to in the food industry as mechanically deboned meat (MDM). I don't know about you, but when I think of the term "mechanically deboned meat," I picture a fancy laser gizmo cutting meat from the bone with machinelike precision. But Wikipedia describes mechanically deboned meat as a pastelike meat product made from forcing pureed chicken under high pressure through a sieve or similar device to separate the bone from the edible meat tissue.* Oh.

When this process is used to create chicken products, the fluoride content can be astronomically high due to residue from chicken bones and other high-fluoride bits that end up in the finished product. In a study published in the *Journal of Agricultural and Food Chemistry,* researchers from Oregon State University measured the fluoride content of various foods made with mechanically separated poultry (Fein and Cerklewski 2001). They found pureed infant foods were highest in fluoride, up to 8.63 ppm, and that a single serving could contain 87 percent of the upper "safe" limit for fluoride for a six-month-old infant (parents beware). Chicken sticks were the next highest, up to 6 ppm, with a single serving providing over 0.5 milligrams of fluoride.

The other two poultry categories they measured, canned meats and luncheon meats, were also high in fluoride, with values as high as 3.65 ppm. Turkey products contain less fluoride than chicken products, but only because the bones are firmer and less likely to end up in the meat. When the researchers measured turkey bones directly, they were found to contain more fluoride than the chicken bones contained, something to keep in mind if you plan on making soup from your Thanksgiving leftovers.

Here is an even dirtier secret dentists will never tell you. Fluoridated drinking water is not the primary reason chicken parts are high in fluoride. Humpty Dumpty had a great fall, indeed.

As we learned in our discussion of California wine, the food and beverage industry (unlike the medical community) has figured out that fluoride is very good at being toxic. According to an EPA ruling from July 15, 2005, the legal limit for fluoride pesticide residue on animal feed is 130 ppm (see "Sulfuryl Fluoride: Pesticide Tolerance"). *One hundred and thirty!* The CDC recommendation for fluoridated drinking water is only 0.7 ppm. The EPA does not have a tolerance for fluoride residue in animal products because they determined "there is

*See https://en.wikipedia.org/wiki/Mechanically_separated_meat

no reasonable expectation of finite residues" (see "Cryolite Summary Document Registration Review"). It appears the EPA does not know how to look up chicken research on PubMed.

Regardless, can you imagine what chicken feed with up to 130 ppm fluoride is doing to their little chicken thyroids and bird-sized pineal glands? Is it absurd to think about chicken thyroids and pineal glands? I think it's absurd not to, but that's just me.*

The studies I've found on the bioaccumulation of fluoride in chickens are focused on chicken bones or mechanically separated meat, but as we've seen with other studies, fluoride can accumulate in tissues other than bone. I've found that my skin does not react to commercially raised chicken breast as long as it is not cooked on the bone, but bone-in chicken, chicken skin, or even a small bite with gristle will cause a fluoroderma reaction if the chicken was not raised to strict organic standards.

I experimented with making chicken soup from a large national brand of organic chicken purchased at the grocery store, but my skin still had a reaction. I suspect either the chicken was provided fluoridated water to drink or perhaps there is some leeway in the organic certification process. I gave up on chicken soup for a few years, but then one Thanksgiving, we purchased a beautiful organic heritage turkey from our local farmer. I couldn't throw out the carcass without first turning it into soup. It made a thick golden broth that gelled like Jell-O when it cooled and did not cause a single breakout on my skin.

Now I eat grilled chicken legs regularly and consume more chicken soup than Jack Canfield's soul.† The key is to purchase organic chicken

---

*"... the pineal gland in birds is located under the skull in the middle of the bird's forehead. The skull in this area is actually thin enough for light to penetrate through the skin and skull bone to directly stimulate the pineal gland, which also has photoreceptors. It is like a third eye. So even a chicken that is blind can still "see the light" and continue to have a relatively normal reproductive system as long as they have the right exposure to light and dark periods." See Elsbeth Upton, "The Avian Pineal Gland: Even a Blind Chicken Can See Spring Coming," *Backyard Poultry,* March 10, 2014.

†See Jack Canfield and Mark Victor Hansen, *Chicken Soup for the Soul* (Deerfield Beach, FL: HCI, 1993).

from a farm you trust. Chicken labeled natural or free-range is not the same as organic. It might still be low in fluoride if the chicken did not drink fluoridated water or eat feed sprayed with fluoride-based pesticides, but you would need to ask the farmer to verify. The organic certification is expensive for small farmers who sometimes raise their chickens to organic standards but can't afford the label. I purchase chicken from the same farmer I found for milk. For more information on how to find a traditional farmer near you, see www.HiddenCauseofAcne.com/food-supply.

If Humpty Dumpty did not convince you as to Lewis Carroll's anti-fluoride subtext in *Alice in Wonderland,* let's talk about the Walrus and the Carpenter for a moment, shall we? What jumps out at you when you think about walruses? It's those two ridiculously long canine teeth that protrude from their upper jaws like elephant tusks, right? You're not going to believe this, but they contain fluoride (National Research Council 1952, 332).

Like birds and humans, marine species bioaccumulate fluoride in their teeth and bones. Researchers have found that the fluoride content of saltwater seems to increase with its salinity (Weinstein and Davison 2004), but it also becomes less bioavailable because of the increased mineral content of water with higher salinity (Camargo 2003). Fluoride in saltwater has a different structure than fluoride in fresh water because of sea water's high magnesium content. Approximately half of the fluoride in sea water is bound with magnesium (Camargo 2003).

While most of us don't eat walrus tusks, some foods do contain fish bones that are high in fluoride. For example, canned salmon often comes packed with the skin and bones. Sardines and anchovies are commonly served whole. The fluoride in seafood is a mystery I have not yet been able to completely figure out. Some sources claim it is caused by environmental pollution, both natural and industrial, while other sources claim all seafood, even protein from fish, is naturally high in fluoride. My skin does not break out from things like fish, shellfish, sea salt, or even seafood bisque, which is prepared by simmering seafood shells in water to make a stock.

At one point I thought perhaps the fluoride in fish bones might not provoke my acne, but I tested this theory to the extreme on a trip to Italy where we dined on the Mediterranean coast at a restaurant with an entire page on the menu devoted to anchovy appetizers. The waiter convinced me to order the "anchovy fantasy platter" to taste a few of their most popular dishes. He brought out a plate of six whole anchovies, perfectly grilled, caught fresh that morning. Then he brought a plate of fried anchovies. Then stuffed. Then marinated. Then things got a little fuzzy, but I know there were more anchovies involved. It was clear by the next morning that anchovies can cause fluoroderma, at least when eaten to excess.

We'll talk more about seafood in chapter 6. For now, just know that avoiding fish bones will help reduce your fluoride exposure. Sorry to break the bad news to all you fish bone lovers out there!

Now about that Carpenter. Carpenters work with the natural grain of wood to transform raw plant parts into finished products that become part of our everyday lives. Isn't it obvious? Carroll is hinting about breakfast cereal there, *duh*. (Get it? Transforming plant parts into stuff we use daily? Never mind.) Grains on their own don't contain significant amounts of fluoride, but extruded breakfast cereals like *puffed* rice, *flaked* corn, and *shredded* wheat often do. The reason is because they are processed with the same type of technique used in the manufacturing of milk solids.

In the production of most commercial breakfast cereals, grains (usually rice, oats, corn, or wheat) are mixed with water, processed into a slurry, and then placed in a machine called an extruder where they are forced through a small hole at a high temperature and pressure, shaping them into stars or whatever shape the picture on the box dictates. When the water from the slurry evaporates, any fluoride it contained is left concentrated in the cereal. One study of cereals processed in fluoridated versus nonfluoridated regions found significant differences in their fluoride content, with cereals processed in fluoridated water ranging from 3.8 to 6.3 ppm (Warren and Levy 2003).

Virtually all boxed breakfast cereals are manufactured with this extrusion process, even "organic" ones found in the health food store. Since the fluoride in water is not a pesticide, it does not count for organic labeling purposes.

You can still eat cereal for breakfast if you have fluoroderma, but the best option is the old-fashioned method of purchasing fresh whole grains and making them yourself. Preparing whole oats might be a little more cumbersome than pouring yourself a bowl of kibble for breakfast, but it's really not that difficult, especially if you set the oats out the night before to soak in an acidic medium (such as water with a spoonful of yogurt, whey, or apple cider vinegar). This was the tradition prior to boxed breakfast cereals coming into fashion and is basically the first step in fermentation, a longstanding traditional process that makes grains and other foods more nutritious and easier to digest.

Oats are just one option. If you've been letting cartoon tigers influence your breakfast decisions, you might be pleasantly surprised by the variety of *real* cereals you've been missing out on. Quinoa, millet, buckwheat, amaranth—these are all just as easy to prepare as oats.

Okay, so the Carpenter and the cereal connection was a stretch. Clearly we're just riding out this *Alice in Wonderland* theme because a) it's fun and b) it's a proven medical fact that antifluoridationists like a good conspiracy theory. While we're at it, we might as well introduce our own character that Lewis Carroll would have included in Wonderland if he really was writing about fluoride.

As you recall, Tweedledumb represents fluoridated water. Tweedledee represents beverages made with fluoridated water. Tweedledodo, the lesser-known brother of Dumb and Dee, represents *food* made with fluoridated water.

Foods that absorb fluoridated water during the cooking process will add to the fluoride load on your skin. Pasta, rice, mashed potatoes, steamed vegetables—these are all potential sources of fluoride because of the water they contain. Think of Tweedledodo as "that guy" who worms his way into a place at your table when you run into him while you're eating out with your friends. For some reason I picture him wearing a T-shirt with a big *F* on it, but of course he's not that obvious about it. Most menus include enough grilled, roasted, or sautéed foods that it is possible to avoid making room for him at your table without looking rude. Salad is usually another safe choice as long as it doesn't contain quinoa or other ingredients made with fluoridated water.

There is one major food source of fluoride we still need to add to our list, and this one is just too weird. Remember the Eat Me cake Alice consumed when she needed a way to grow taller so she could reach the golden key for the door leading from the bottom of the rabbit hole into the Wonderland garden? As Carroll describes, it was a little cake "on which the words 'Eat Me' were beautifully marked in currants." Because I lived in Scotland, I know this one: currants is the British code word for *raisins*. (You should let that one sink in for a moment.)

Raisins are high in fluoride for the same reason some wine is high in fluoride. Virtually all raisins in the United States are grown in the central San Joaquin Valley or, as Western Grapeleaf Skeletonizers and Omnivorous Leafrollers refer to it, the Promised Land.

The USDA data sheet for fluoride lists raisins at 2.34 ppm, but as we've seen with other foods, those numbers have so many variables that putting stock in a government average is like taking the Queen of Hearts's facial impressions at face value. Researchers at the University of Kansas measured five brands of California raisins and found fluoride levels as high as 5.2 ppm (Burgstahler and Robinson 1997). However, there is reason to believe that if you play raisin roulette long enough, you will stumble onto some raisins with much more fluoride than that.

The amount of fluoride in raisins depends on a number of factors including the quantity of pesticide used, the rate of dilution, timing of the application, humidity levels, rainfall, war rations, a government-sanctioned raisin mafia that could only exist in Wonderland, and current trends in baked goods.

As you can probably tell, there's a story here. It is reaching from beyond the grave to be told, barking at me to assume the role of storyteller with an insistence I can't refuse. So grab a fluoride-free drink and a raisin-free snack, dim the lights, and settle in for what it sure to be a twisted tale as I present to you: the untold story of raisins.

> *Humpty Dumpty sat on a wall,*
> *Bones of fluoride—skin, joints, and all.*
> *Awful fish carcass, Tweedledodo said,*
> *Let's poison cereal with raisins instead.*

IMPOSSIBLE THINGS AT BREAKFAST

The story of American raisins begins in the late nineteenth century when advancements in irrigation and railroad transportation enabled large-scale commercial raisin production in California. In 1912, raisin growers in Fresno formed the California Associated Raisin Company, chaired by H. H. Welsh, and launched their first marketing campaign two years later during the outbreak of World War I. Raisin prices sky-rocketed during the war as the military purchased them as cheap snacks for troops. European allies imported California raisins by the boatload thanks to credits from the U.S. Food Administration. Boiled raisin cakes known as "war cakes," made without milk or eggs, became a sym-bol of American resourcefulness and were sent in care packages to troops overseas. Raisin production increased during the war to meet demand, but farmers were devastated after the war when prices plummeted.

The demand for raisins surged again in the 1940s, this time in the face of the Nazi threat. In 1942, the War Production Board ordered California's entire wine grape crop be made into raisins. Raisin vineyard acreage expanded as prices soared from $48 per ton in 1939 to $312 per ton in 1946. Things really got serious when mock mincemeat pies filled with raisins replaced regular mincemeat pies filled with whatever regular mincemeat pies are filled with.

This time when the war ended, the government was ready with a foolproof plan—or so they thought. Raisin farmers would continue to grow absurd amounts of raisins, but to keep prices high, they would only be allowed to sell a portion of their crops. The rest would be seized by the government and squirreled away in raisin bunkers for a rainy day world war. Or they would be sold to foreigners at low prices to devastate raisin farmers overseas. At the very least, they would be fed to disappointed schoolchildren and confused cows. It was an ingenious idea. What could go wrong?

The plan was implemented in 1949 as part of the New Deal when the U.S. Department of Agriculture created the National Raisin Reserve. Instead of selling raisins directly on the free market, U.S. raisin growers began shipping their raisins to a raisin "handler" who separated the raisins due the federal government and paid the grower only for the remainder. Technically, raisin growers were supposed to receive a share of profits made on the sale of reserve raisins, but even during years when they generated $65 million in sales, there was nothing left over to share with raisin farmers who, for the most part, were happy they didn't have to think up their own raisin commercials and were content with the inflated prices they were receiving on the domestic market.

Speaking of raisin commercials, you might remember this part of the story. At the height of the raisin cartel glory days, a government grant of $3 million was provided to help boost sales abroad by partially funding a marketing campaign about a raisin claymation musical group called the California Raisins, who released four studio albums, starred in their own Saturday morning cartoon show, were featured in an Emmy award-winning Christmas special, and were permanently enshrined in the National Museum of American History. Meanwhile in the target market of Japan, where no one bothered to translate the commercials into Japanese, viewers mistook the singing raisins for chocolate candy or potatoes (White 2009). The campaign eventually ran into legal trouble when California raisin farmers argued the advertisements cost almost twice what the California producers were earning from extra raisins sold in Japan.

As good as the idea of a national raisin reserve sounds, the cache never came in as handy as government officials must have thought it would. And yet, the reserve persisted until June 2015 when the U.S. Supreme Court sided with a stubborn farmer named Marvin Horne who refused to let the government seize his raisins.

"This is an interesting story, Melissa, but what does it have to do with fluoride?" My goodness, can't a woman write about raisins for a few hundred words anymore? I haven't even made any raisin' puns yet, or clever plays on the words grapes and wrath.

As I was *about to say,* now that you know the story behind California raisins, you can see that well-intentioned government policy has been causing the overproduction of raisins in California for generations. This explains the longtime mystery of why raisins are given out as healthy treats at Halloween instead of personal-sized packets of dehydrated apples, pineapple, or papaya, to give just a few examples (hint, hint). It also explains why in America, raisins are seen as "the cool, hip dried fruit for kids" while prunes, which are basically just big raisins, are used solely to deconstipate old people. Raisins are the most popular dried fruit in the United States, accounting for approximately two-thirds of total dried fruit consumption. That's not fair. The story of California raisins also shows how the United States grew to become the largest exporter of raisins in the world, exporting to nearly fifty countries and producing almost half of the world's raisin supply—all from within a 60-mile radius of Fresno.

Here is where the full-grown gorilla takes the stage. When large plots of land are used to grow a single crop like this, year after year, farming experts refer to it as monocropping. Over time, monocrops become more difficult to protect as nature intervenes in an attempt to restore biodiversity to the region. This is why grape growers in San Joaquin Valley need to rely on a toxic fluoride-based pesticide like cryolite to control Western Grapeleaf Skeletonizers and Omnivorous Leafrollers while vineyard workers in other parts of California don't need to use pesticides at all and have never even heard of cryolite.

The California Department of Pesticide Regulation (CDPR)

describes cryolite as one of a few "widely applied insecticides" commonly used in the state. In 2013 alone, over half a million pounds of cryolite were applied to California farmland, most of it in the self-described raisin capital of the world, San Joaquin Valley.* The EPA previously set a blanket tolerance for fluoride residue at 7 ppm but has since lifted the tolerance for certain food crops in response to petitions from the same cryolite manufacturers who successfully petitioned to increase the European limit for fluoride in California wine.

Reading about cryolite tolerances got me wondering about who monitors and enforces all these pesticide regulations. It's all well and good to have tolerances for pesticide residue, but is that like a strict mafia rule, e.g. "deliver this package or you'll swim with the fishes"? Or is it more like a strict librarian rule, e.g. "bring back this book or I'll fine you five cents per day"?

As it turns out, it's neither. The EPA is only responsible for establishing the tolerances for pesticide residue. The monitoring and enforcement aspect is left to the Food and Drug Administration and the Department of Agriculture. According to the most recent annual summary report for the FDA's pesticide monitoring program, the FDA uses measuring methods that detect 484 various pesticides. Cryolite is not on the list.[†]

Cryolite is the third most used pesticide on the second most productive crop in the number one agricultural producing state in the country. Why is the FDA not monitoring for it?

Even more incredible, according to the online FDA database for domestic food products, the FDA rarely inspects California raisins for any pesticide residue whatsoever. In 2012, for example, the FDA did not perform a single test for pesticide residue on the undefeated dried fruit champion of the American food scene. Meanwhile domestic craisins, raisins' sworn archenemy, were inspected for 380 different pesticides.

---

*To sleuth around California's pesticide databases, visit http://www.cdpr.ca.gov
†To sleuth around the FDA's pesticide monitoring databases, visit https://www.fda.gov/Food/FoodborneIllnessContaminants/Pesticides

Imported raisins are a different story. In 2012, the FDA inspected raisins from Afghanistan, Argentina, Canada, Chile, China, and South Africa. The United States only imports a teensy portion of the 220,000 metric tons of raisins consumed by Americans each year. Why is the FDA focused on inspecting raisins imported from Canada and neglecting California raisins? And how did they even find raisins imported from Canada? That's like looking for a craisin in a raisin bunker.

The Department of Agriculture and California State labs don't test for cryolite either. Like the FDA, they seem to have stopped the routine monitoring of domestic raisins for pesticide residue in the 1990s. To give you an idea of how strange this is, in an average year, let's go with 2011, the California Department of Pesticide Regulation tested for pesticide residue on 24 jicama, 23 chayote, 6 watercress, 3 water chestnuts, and 0 raisins. According to their sampling history database, they inspect other common fruits and vegetables like oranges, eggplant, cantaloupe, garlic, and raspberries every year. But raisins, for the most part, have had a free pass. Could that have anything to do with the government-sanctioned raisin mafia, or the $5 billion California vineyards bring in as revenue each year? With the exception of almonds, that's more money than any other food crop in California.

I don't know why California stopped routinely inspecting raisins for pesticides in 1989, but I do know this: the country that produces half the world's raisin supply from one monocrop outside of Fresno barely monitors them for pesticides.

Speaking of 1989, that happened to be the same year wine-sniffing Europeans noticed excessive amounts of fluoride in the California wine they were importing. As Charlotte Means noted in a 2002 report from the ASPCA's Animal Poison Control Center, 1989 also marked the beginning of a trend in dogs who confiscated cartons of raisins from the pantries of their live-in house servants. Within hours, the dogs developed vomiting, diarrhea, and in some cases, lethal kidney failure. *These are all symptoms of acute fluoride poisoning, people.*

While California pesticide regulators were busy in the 1990s inspecting cherimoya and celeriac, raisin toxicity in dogs continued to be reported in cases throughout the world and across a variety of brands consumed, which should not have been surprising considering half the world's raisin supply, regardless of brand, is produced from the same monocrop in California. ASPCA veterinarians claim pesticides are an unlikely cause of raisin toxicity in dogs, but as we've seen before, health care professionals in the United States have a blind spot to the adverse health effects of fluoride. Let's take a closer look at their supporting evidence.

In a 2005 study published in the *Journal of Veterinary Internal Medicine,* veterinary toxicologist Paul Eubig and his colleagues from the ASPCA's Animal Poison Control Center conducted a retrospective analysis of forty-three cases of acute renal failure in dogs following the ingestion of raisins and grapes. The earliest case report included in the study was from 1992 (a year California raisin growers dropped over two million pounds of cryolite on their raisin crops). Veterinarians think of themselves as dog specialists, so they focused on the dog part of the story, which explains why most of the retrospective study is an intensely close and personal look at dog pee. But now that you've read my raisin saga, I think it's safe to say that you and I are armchair raisin specialists. So we are going to focus on the raisins.

Of the 43 dogs in the study, 28 ingested raisins, 13 ingested grapes, and 2 ingested both. In 13 of the cases, Labrador retrievers played the leading part of raisin thief with 19 other breeds making up the remainder.* Only 23 of the dogs survived their grape/raisin snack, and 8 of the surviving dogs experienced long-term side effects.

The dosage of raisins the dogs consumed ranged anywhere from

---

*Clearly Labrador retrievers are more susceptible to raisin poisoning because they figured out the secret to life, happiness, and everything is the more you retrieve, the more you can eat and the more you eat, the more you can retrieve. This theory is confirmed by the ten-year-old yellow Labrador retriever sitting by my side as I write this book. If I brought raisins into the house, she would most certainly confiscate them. Her name is Gia. She says hi.

2.8 to 19.6 grams per kilogram of body weight.* The veterinary toxicologists found this odd. Generally, when a substance is toxic, the more of it you consume, the more likely you are to become sick. The ASPCA researchers hypothesized that the lack of a dose-response relationship might be due to an extrinsic substance that is not always present on raisins, but they quickly discounted pesticides as a likely culprit because they reasoned any pesticide residue would not contain high enough concentrations to cause renal failure. What evidence do they provide to support this claim? The veterinarians point to FDA inspections of domestic table grapes (not raisins) from 2002 in which twenty samples of the six million tons of California grapes produced that year were found to be perfectly safe. Of course you and I know those samples weren't even tested for residue from the millions of pounds of toxic cryolite dumped over California.

The other evidence the ASPCA veterinarians cite was from one of the dog case studies where the offending raisins were tested for chlorinated hydrocarbon, carbamate, and organophosphorus insecticides. If even a single Raisin 101 class was taught in the school system these days, the veterinarians would have known to test for fluoride too. But because our society is largely raisin-illiterate, the opportunity was wasted.

I admit the story of fluoride and raisins sounds like an impossible thing to believe about a dried fruit you sprinkle on your breakfast cereal. When did we fall down a raisin chute and end up in Willy Wonka's Mad Hatter Raisin Factory? I might be mixing my Johnny Depp metaphors here, but you know what I mean. Could the EPA, the FDA, the USDA, and the entire state of California all be conspiring on such an expansive plot?

Here's how this works. It's not that our government is full of evil bureaucrats who congregate in cubicles, plotting ways to poison the rest of the population. I observed government workers in their native habitat

---

*In a 2008 article in the *Daily Mail* entitled "Massive increase in dogs poisoned by chocolate and grapes fed to them by their owners," Rebecca Camber notes dogs have died from eating as few as four grapes.

long enough to know this is not the norm. Most government employees are good people, even dentists, and they just want to show up, get the job done (with minimal effort, let's be honest), and go home to their families. Government bureaucrats tend to be more risk averse than your average American entrepreneur. This trait, along with their propensity to use Microsoft Word's cut-and-paste feature (or until very recently, WordPerfect), means the status quo is almost always favored. Why rewrite the wheel when you can submit the same old wheel everyone else has been wheeling since 1945? Rewriting wheels is risky business, and government bureaucrats a) don't do risk and b) don't do business. They do bureaucracy.

It is statistically probable that outright corruption goes on from time to time. Have *you* ever tried to refuse an offer from the raisin mafia? But in my experience here in the United States, bad things happen mainly because bureaucrats are just normal people behaving as normal people tend to behave, with a few rotten raisins thrown in the mix.

Take for example the government's efforts to regulate cryolite. Even though it was first approved in 1957, EPA evaluators admitted decades later that their database for cryolite was still "extremely poor" with "extensive data gaps" in all disciplines. When the EPA reregistered cryolite in 1996, the pesticide was a forty-year incumbent. That's a lot of quo for a government bureaucrat to overcome. And this wasn't your generic "we always do it this way" brand of status quo. By 1996, cryolite had a rare vintage of hyper quo that pesticides like DDT never dreamed possible. This is where we see the fingerprints of our story's biggest villains, despite their careful use of latex gloves.

Since cryolite is basically just ground fluoride minerals, the EPA treats it as fluoride. As a result, all the work that dentists and the devil did over the past century to try to prove that fluoride added to the water supply is "safe and effective" was used to vouch for the safety of cryolite too. The EPA evaluators who reregistered cryolite readily admit that it accumulates in the body at all doses, but they don't consider that a bad thing. When one of the studies in their review suggested that "severe maternal toxicity" occurs at lower cryolite doses, the EPA simply deemed the study unacceptable. Their justification was copied and pasted directly from a government review on fluoridated water.*

The EPA reregistration decision is overflowing with overlooked warning signs of cryolite's toxicity. To give one last example, one of the studies the EPA used to evaluate the safety of cryolite was from Battelle Laboratory. The lab was tasked with conducting a study on baby Easter bunnies to gauge the safety of cryolite when it comes into contact with the skin. When several "diva" bunnies died after licking their fur—an act that was not in their contract—EPA told Battelle not to bother with a do-over since cryolite was already known to be safe when applied topically. Despite the "extreme sensitivity of the rabbit to oral doses of cryolite," the EPA went on to approve the use of cryolite on the food we feed our children, our dogs, and occasionally, our rabbits.

CATERPILLARS BLOWING SMOKE

The food and beverages described in this chapter so far are the common sources of fluoride I came across during my experience of fluoroderma, but I would not be surprised if your list is different. You and I live on different pieces of earth. We eat diverse foods and breathe distant air. It is entirely possible you will run into sources of fluoride I have not yet encountered. In those situations, you will need to do your own investigative work. But you already have access to all the resources any superhero needs to be successful: a nerdy sidekick like Internet and a superpower (your little layman brain).†

For example, raisins are all the rage right now, but perhaps you, being the enlightened raisin rebel that you now are, develop an affinity for dried apricots instead. *Viva la resistance!* If you ask Internet if

---

*For a haunting read, visit www.HiddenCauseofAcne.com/resources to view the EPA's Reregistration Eligibility Decision for cryolite.

†Since *layman* is a relative term, ALL of us have brains that are mostly layman (with maybe a little nonlayman mixed in).

cryolite can be used on apricots, she will take you to the EPA database for pesticide tolerances that confirms, as with grapes, fresh apricots have a residue tolerance for fluoride of 7 ppm. Does that mean dried apricots are high in fluoride? I don't know. Maybe? Sometimes? Not really? You will have to look at where your apricot stash is produced and then research pesticide usage reports for that region. Or contact the manufacturer. Or do some experiments on your skin to see how it reacts. Or just eat organic apricots instead.

The use of cryolite is not restricted to California and it's not reserved for dried fruit. Cryolite is allowed to be applied to a variety of crops throughout the United States, including lettuce, berries, brussels sprouts, eggplant, kale, peaches, peppers, plums, tomatoes, and more.* My fluoroderma convinced me to switch to organic produce and therefore I do not have extensive experience on whether or not any of these foods cause breakouts. I still eat what I assume to be conventional produce at most restaurants. As long as they aren't steamed in fluoridated water, my skin doesn't seem to mind.

Fields, orchards, and vineyards aren't the only places fluoridated chemical warfare is waged in the name of mass produce. In the last decade, another avenue for fluoride-based pesticides has risen to the forefront of the American food supply. The story begins with the return of everyone's favorite story-time character: raisins.

If you've ever seen the inside of a raisin warehouse, you know exactly what I am talking about. Whole species of invaders have risen up in San Joaquin Valley to seize humanity's hard-fought heaps of raisin booty. Dusky raisin moths, hairy fungus beetles, bark lice—these are just a few of the callous warriors caught looting our rightful raisin caches. They covertly infiltrate our bunkers while the Raisin Reserves are sleeping, setting up shanty towns that attract predators of their own. To facilitate their mission of carrying off dying larvae of

*For a map of cryolite use in the United States, see the cryolite page of the National Water Quality Program's Pesticide National Synthesis Project created by the U.S. Geological Survey at www.HiddenCauseofAcne.com/resources

storage moths stung by parasites, dedicated armies of brown ants dig impressive underground tunnel systems extending to depths of 3 feet or more. In springtime, surviving larvae pupate and emerge from the raisin depths.*

To combat enemy forces, in 2002, raisin handlers started using a toxic gas called ProFume to fumigate raisin warehouses. You are probably unfamiliar with ProFume unless you work in the industry, but you might know its older sibling, Vikane. Since the early 1960s, Vikane has been the cornerstone of residential termite fumigation and is also occasionally used to control bedbugs and other infestations. Both Vikane and ProFume were developed by Dow AgroSciences using sulfuryl fluoride as the active ingredient.

As with cryolite, EPA considers fluoride as the toxicological endpoint of concern with sulfuryl fluoride, but unlike cryolite, there is no confusion over the fact that sulfuryl fluoride is highly toxic to humans. Even dentists can't find a way to dismiss the health effects experienced by people like Peyton McCaughey, a ten-year-old boy in South Florida, who in 2015 suffered extensive brain damage after returning to his house, which was recently fumigated with sulfuryl fluoride to kill termites (Ganim 2015).

Despite its known toxicity, the EPA approved the use of sulfuryl fluoride on food products in 2002 with an Experimental Use Permit that allowed 12 ppm for fluoride on walnuts and 30 ppm on raisins. (Dow had petitioned for an exemption to the requirement for a fluoride tolerance on raisins, but EPA's Mathematics Department calculated 30 ppm as a fair compromise between 12 and infinity.) The United States needed an alternative to methyl bromide, another pesticide Dow produced, which was globally banned by the Vienna Convention's

---

*"During one harvest, a beetle of the family Curculionidae, *Dinocleus capillosus* Csiki, was abundant in vineyards and later in the boxed raisins. The insects were about the same size and weight as seedless raisins. Raisin-cleaning machinery did not remove them; expensive hand-sorting was necessary." See U.S. Department of Agriculture, "Insects on Dried Fruit, Agriculture Handbook 464" (Simmons and Nelson 1975, 9).

Montreal Protocol. If you refer back to our handy periodic chart from chapter 3, you'll notice that bromine sits below fluorine in the halogen group. After learning their lesson with methyl bromide, most countries at least made an attempt to pursue less toxic pesticides in its place. But not in the United States. We decided to spray our snacks with termite fumigant instead.

In 2004, just two years after the Experimental Use Permit was approved for raisins and walnuts, sulfuryl fluoride was approved for widespread use as a food fumigant. Consequently, EPA set the highest levels of fluoride residue ever allowed on food in the United States, including 70 ppm for beans, 125 ppm for wheat flour, and *900* ppm for powdered eggs. At that point, why not just make scrambled eggs out of sodium fluoride powder? (This does not end well.)* Or eat a toothpaste sandwich?†

Consumer protection groups like the Fluoride Action Network, the Environmental Working Group, and Beyond Pesticides joined forces with a pro bono lawyer from American University to try to reverse EPA's approval of sulfuryl fluoride as a food fumigant. In 2011, after eight years of effort, EPA was forced to admit that children were overexposed to aggregate sources of fluoride. By their own calculations, they estimated that sulfuryl fluoride accounted for 3 percent of total fluoride exposure, and thus they agreed to phase it out over a period of three years.

Realizing EPA was trapped by ineffable algorithms from its own Mathematics Department, Dow switched its focus to Congressional lobbies and managed to slip a sentence into President Obama's 1,000-page Farm Bill ordering EPA without explanation to ignore all nonpesticide

---

*In 1942, a cook at Oregon State Hospital for the Insane made scrambled eggs for 467 mental patients using sodium fluoride (used for rat poison at the asylum) instead of powdered milk. It was an honest mistake, but 47 of the patients died by the next day. (John 2012).

†See www.HiddenCauseofAcne.com/Al-Bundy-toothpaste-sandwich (do not try this at home)

sources of fluoride when calculating fluoride pesticide tolerances.* The sentence was added just a few days before the final vote, leaving little time for the public to organize opposition or for government politicians to understand what they were signing. Of course that did not keep them from signing it.

When Obama proudly signed the Farm Bill into law in February 2014, the United States became one of only two countries that allows sulfuryl fluoride to be sprayed on food (see "The Universal Consensus on Sulfuryl Fluoride = Keep It Away from Food" 2013). With their market share safely intact, the Dow Chemical Company then offloaded Dow AgroSciences, the division that produces Vikane and ProFume, in a sale to Douglas Products one year later. A Dow spokesperson claimed the reason for the sale was because the company "believes that this business segment has a greater opportunity to reach its full potential under a different owner. [And also, did you see what we just went through to get that sh** approved? Buy low, sell high, hold through tough times. Duh.]"†

With government actors writing the rules (as industry lobbyists whisper them their lines), it's easy to feel demoralized, disillusioned, and defeated. But let's not focus on them. Let's focus on *you*. You don't need to be a victim of the government's delusional approach to raisin-inspired chemical warfare. If the idea of eating termite fumigant does not appeal to you, you have the option of buying organic. That probably means you

---

*"Notwithstanding any other provision of law, the Administrator of the Environmental Protection Agency shall exclude nonpesticidal sources of fluoride from any aggregate exposure assessment required under section 408 of the Federal Food, Drug, and Cosmetic Act (21 U.S.C. 346a) when assessing tolerances associated with residues from the pesticide." See "Regulation of Sulfuryl Fluoride" H.R. 2642, Public Law No. 113–79, Section 10015, https://www.congress.gov/bill/113th-congress/house-bill/2642/text?overview=closed

†If you haven't figured this out yet, I am a hyperquoter. It's a medical condition that results in a chemical compulsion to insert sass when called for, even if it means breaking the accepted rules of grammar. I wouldn't call it misquoting, though, it's more like quoting between the lines. If you missed the May 8 edition of *Pest Control Technology*, then you can read the original boring quote here: Brad Harbison, "Dow to Sell Sulfuryl Fluoride to Douglas Products," *Pest Control Technology*, May 8, 2015.

will need to spend more money and might even have to change your shopping venues, but once you understand the health risk associated with raisin roulette—and produce poker in general—it is easier to find room in your budget.

When I first realized the negative effect fluoride was causing on my skin, I did not have a job and I was in debt from an upside-down mortgage for a house I could not live in. Organic food seemed needlessly expensive compared to what I was accustomed to buying, but my cystic acne was strong motivation to change my shopping habits. I watched basic cable on a 13-inch hand-me-down television and used a flip phone long after iPhones hit the market, but I managed to buy organic food because it was my priority. If you suffer from cystic acne like I did, and have money to buy books to indulge your guilty obsession with raisin dramas, then I suspect organic food will be a priority for you too—especially now that you're privy to the long-concealed secret that diet causes acne (and sometimes other bad side effects, like death).

There are a few other sources of fluoride exposure you might run into besides diet. Pesticide manufacturers have discovered that fluoride is good at killing unwanted house guests, but it has many other utilities. As I mentioned in chapter 1, fluoride can alter the melting point of metals. It can also make chemicals more durable, modify their propensity to dissolve in fats and oils, or increase the bioavailability of pharmaceuticals by enabling more of the dose to reach systemic circulation.

Approximately 20 percent of pharmaceuticals are estimated to contain fluoride, including many of the top drugs such as Prozac, Paxil, Cipro, Flonase, and Lipitor to name just a few (Thayer 2006).* According to Manfred Schlosser, a professor of chemistry at the Swiss Federal Institute of Technology, a rule of thumb in medicinal chemistry is that "smuggling fluorine into a lead structure enhances the probability of landing a hit almost 10-fold" (Thayer 2006).

Drug manufacturers will tell you this type of fluoride is so sta-

---

*For a more comprehensive list, see www.slweb.org/ftrcfluorinatedpharm.html

ble it does not break down in the human body, and yet some studies clearly show elevated levels of fluoride in urine or blood following the use of fluoridated medication (Rimoli et al. 1991; Pradhan et al. 1995; "Sources of Fluoride: Pharmaceuticals" n.d.).

Speaking of unintended bodily consequences, remember the Scotchgard debacle, when we realized the chemical 3M was marketing to save seat cushions from wine stains wasn't just accumulating in human tissue but could also be found in arctic polar bears who didn't care about their seat cushions and rarely even drink wine?* Fluoride was the culprit at that crime scene. Over a decade after banning the Scotchgard formula, we are still trying to figure out what exactly is going on with those fluoridated chemicals after they enter living bodies and how to clean them up.

Perhaps you are familiar with the controversy surrounding nonstick cookware? Yes, the f-word is to blame there too. The same super-strong fluoride bonds that keep wine from adhering to seat cushions also prevent other national emergencies such as eggs sticking to pans. As their own internal documents attest, DuPont, the makers of Teflon, noticed as early as 1955 that "harmful compounds" were given off in the air when their nonstick pans were heated above 400 degrees Fahrenheit. They didn't bother telling anyone about it at the time because they were not able to "duplicate in animal tests *the symptoms observed in humans*" (emphasis added because *really?!*).†

Besides releasing harmful contents into the air, nonstick coating can also add fluoride to the cooking contents. A study published in the *Journal of Dental Research* measured the fluoride content of water that had been boiled for fifteen minutes in pots made of aluminum, stainless

---

*I say "rarely" because of this guy: www.thedrinksbusiness.com/2015/11/polar-bear-raids -bbc-film-crew-wine-supply

†"Two types of reaction have been noted in humans as the result of accidental inhalation of the products of heated polymer. 1) a condition similar to metal fever; and 2) a condition in which there may be an irritation of the lungs leading to pulmonary edema." See DuPont bulletin No. X-59a, as quoted in Bryson 2011, kindle location 7809.

steel, pyrex, and Teflon (Full and Parkins 1975). The water boiled in Teflon contained three times more fluoride than any of the other samples.

DuPont first recognized the commercial potential of fluoride bonds when they created refrigerants by combining fluoride, chlorine, and carbon into a chemical known as chloro*fluoro*carbons (CFCs). CFCs were used in aerosol cans, fire extinguishers, cleaning solvents, and other products. They were eventually banned by the Montreal Protocol because of their detrimental effect on the ozone layer; however, they were largely replaced by hydro*fluoro*carbons (which still contain fluoride) and had already spawned an entire catalogue of other fluoride-based chemicals. In addition to nonstick cookware and stain protectors, fluoride is still used in an assortment of products such as flame retardants, cosmetics, waterproof clothing, greasy food packaging, pizza boxes, and microwave popcorn bags.

In May 2015, hundreds of scientists from around the world signed a document called the Madrid Statement published in *Environmental Health Perspectives* to warn of the severe health risks associated with the promiscuous use of fluorinated chemicals and to call for their restricted use and further study (Blum et al. 2015). In a response published in the same journal issue and written by a lawyer from the FluoroCouncil, a global organization representing the world's leading fluorotechnology companies, the industry admits the old fluoride chemicals they sold us for the last fifty plus years were really bad and should definitely be removed from production, but they assure us the new and improved fluoride chemicals they are planning to sell us for the next fifty plus years are "less toxic" and remain in living tissue and the atmosphere for "substantially shorter" periods of time (Bowman 2015).*

---

*To read the scientists' response to the FluoroCouncil's statement, see Ian Cousins et al., "Comment on 'Fluorotechnology Is Critical to Modern Life: The FluoroCouncil Counterpoint to the Madrid Statement,'" *Environmental Health Perspectives* 123, no. 7 (2015), http://ehp.niehs.nih.gov/1510207. To read the FluoroCouncil's response to their response, see Jessica Bowman, "Response to 'Comment on "Fluorotechnology Is Critical to Modern Life: The FluoroCouncil Counterpoint to the Madrid Statement,"'" *Environmental Health Perspectives* 123, no. 7 (2015), http://ehp.niehs.nih.gov/1510295.

It's a tough call, but I say we go with the global community of independent scientists on this one.

Realizing our modern lives are set in a piping hot bowl of toxic suey causes some people (*Dad!*) to throw up their hands in defeat. "Something's gotta kill you eventually," they reason, "so you might as well eat poisoned popcorn." That's stupid. Don't do that. Unpoisoned popcorn is tastier anyway.* Other people roll their eyes at the word *toxin* and say things like "If toxins scare you, stop eating."† Very helpful, thanks.

We live in an era when we know enough about chemistry to be dangerous but not enough to be wise. Most of us think someone out there is testing and regulating the safety of the manufactured chemicals staring back at us from the store shelves. We read product labels on carefully designed boxes and assume they tell the whole story, or at least the important parts. The reality is that the legislation regulating industrial chemicals in the United States, known as the Toxic Substances Control Act or TSCA (pronounced "tosca"), was passed into law in 1976 and was not substantially updated for the next *forty years*.

A lot of things changed during that time period. For starters, over half the current U.S. population was born, including me. The EPA banned asbestos because it causes cancer in humans and then unbanned asbestos because it causes lawsuits from industry attorneys. Polar bears settled with 3M for an undisclosed sum of sticky notes in exchange for their continued silence on the Scotchgard incident. CFCs, PCBs, PFOAs, PFOSs—all these acronyms represent lessons we could have been using to improve our approach to industrial chemical regulation.

---

*Here's how to make my favorite homemade popcorn. Heat a generous spoonful of coconut oil in a large pot or a stovetop popcorn maker. Add 3 kernels of organic popcorn and cover the pot. When the kernels pop, add a ½ cup of kernels to the heated oil. Shake the pan or rotate the popcorn turner as the rest of the kernels pop. Sprinkle with sea salt and drench in melted butter from pastured cows. Snuggle on couch and watch *Food, Inc.* or *Elf*, as appropriate for the season.

†Hank Campbell. November 26, 2013. "Thanksgiving Chemophobia: If Toxins Scare You, Stop Eating." *Science 2.0* (blog), http://www.science20.com/science_20/thanksgiving_chemophobia_if_toxins_scare_you_stop_eating-118737

Instead, we kept doing it the same old way we had been doing it since 1976. That's government status quo in inaction. Again.

Our paralysis in chemical regulation goes back even further than the 1970s. When government bureaucrats implemented the Toxic Substances Control Act, they decided to grandfather in 62,000 pre-existing industrial chemicals solely in the name of status quo—most of them were never even tested for adverse health effects. As a result, when you use a common household product to *freshen* air, *soften* fabric, *dissolve* stains, and so on, you are likely relying on the scientific sophistication of a 1950s businessman to guarantee your safety and the marketing prowess of the 1950s adman he hired to inculcate the need for the product deep into your psyche.

If you are accustomed to picking any product off the shelf and giving it a try, then this information should have a dramatic effect on your purchasing habits. But I know it can be hard to rewire your thought process when all these products seem perfectly normal. It's like when I tried to convince my parents they shouldn't trust email from random strangers (or phone calls, *Mom!*) and then visit the websites they suggest. Things might seem fine at the time, but chances are some nasty code made its way into your system, or worse, and your error in judgment will eventually catch up with you. The same is true with our naive trust in industrial chemicals, except when the time comes you won't be able to dump your body's old operating system and switch to a Mac.

To be fair to my parents, everyone succumbs to naïveté in one form or another. Our brains simply weren't designed to rethink every wheel we come across. That's the beauty of technology and human society in general, but it can also limit us to the widely accepted beliefs of the time. To help smooth things over with my parents, I'll give an example from my own collection of dumb things I've done.

One year, my unit at FBI Headquarters was moved to a different office, and everyone was cleaning the Hoover-era crud from their new cubicles. A few times a day, I heard a loud *psssssst* coming from my coworkers' cubes. I eventually figured out they were using cans of "compressed air" to clean between the keys on their keyboards. I had never heard of such an invention, but I thought, "Golly gee, Mr. Businessman, a can of crisp mountain air to dislodge the cookie crumbs inside the crevices of my keyboard? Gee whiz, thanks! What will you come up with next?" As I pulled the trigger, my wide-eyed wonder quickly dissipated when the can turned ice cold in my hand. *Huh?* What kind of white witch cleaning devilry is this? Plain air doesn't do *that*.

Later that evening, Internet hooked me up with a keyboard cleaning data sheet written by two smarty-pants' named Shirli and Larry who work for the City of Seattle. They patiently explained to me that "compressed air" isn't a bottled ocean breeze that propels itself onward full of nothing but sea scent and miracles. The brand of keyboard cleaner we were using was composed of a hydro*fluoro*carbon called HFC-152a. The fluoride-based chemical is also used as a refrigerant, which explains why the can turned cold when I pressed the trigger. According to Shirli and Larry, HFC-152a is a flammable greenhouse gas and causes central nervous system depression leading to headaches and fatigue.

Eureka! Shirli and Larry had hit on something. As my coworkers were diligently tidying up their personal corners of Hoover Heaven, many of them started complaining of headaches, depressed immunity, and poor ventilation in our new workspace. An inspector was assigned to assess if the room was up to code. What are the chances he tested for hydrofluorocarbon? I gave Shirli and Larry's data sheet to my government point of contact, but he just put it with the other papers in the papers-to-be-routed-to-the-routing-box box. I am still waiting to hear back about it. Not long afterward, my team was moved to a new unit in our original workspace (this was not unusual given the government's well-known fondness for a rousing round of musical chairs—*so fun!* Even Shirli likes it).

Like my coworkers, I too experienced headaches while working in the new office before my childlike preconceptions of canned air were crushed, convincing me to find a way to be absent from my workspace until I was officially moved to a new desk. I don't recall hydrofluorocarbon affecting my acne, but I don't know what my skin would look like if I continued to inadvertently sniff chemical keyboard cleaner on a daily basis or if I lived next to an "air" factory.

I am bringing up the topic of fluoridated chemicals not because I have the answers but because you and I need to be asking the questions, instead of relying on 1950s businessmen and EPA's Question Department. Congress finally passed legislation to revise TSCA in 2016, but the products we encounter today were produced under the original TSCA regulations. Under those rules, EPA had ninety days to decide if a new chemical posed an "unreasonable risk" to public health, otherwise the product moved on to the marketing teams for an expert makeover before batting its eyelashes at you from retail shelves. The requisite catch-22 built into the regulatory process was that companies were not required to test their new chemicals, and EPA regulators did not have the resources to do it themselves. Unless a company volunteered to test their chemicals and then provided derogatory information about them to the EPA, the new chemical did not trigger the EPA's initial threshold for testing. So as long as there was no testing, there was no reason for further testing.

The revised TSCA legislation passed in 2016 made comprehensive changes to the existing law, but it remains to be seen how the new regulations will be implemented.* If we don't want to be collateral damage in the meantime, we will need to be discerning consumers instead. Good thing we've been exercising our little layman brains for just such a challenge.

The government's policy has been that industrial chemicals are innocent until proven guilty, but that doesn't mean it has to be our policy too. Unless a chemical product has a solid track record of—I don't know, let's say a few hundred years—then I think it's only prudent based on historical experience to be a little skeptical of it. Your side-

---

*For more information on the revisions made to TSCA, see "Passing a Strong New Chemical Safety Law" by the Environmental Defense Fund at https://www.edf.org /health/policy/chemicals-policy-reform

kick Internet is happy to provide more information on any products you care to ask her about. The Environmental Working Group is an excellent resource for consumer safety information on cleaning products, fire retardants, and other chemical products commonly encountered in our modern lives. Internet will even arrange for healthier options to be shipped directly to your doorstep by connecting you with online retailers who specialize in household products that are typically safer than the ones at Walmart and less expensive than the ones at Whole Foods.

In many cases, you probably don't even need a chemical product to fulfill the task at hand. To demonstrate, Shirli and Larry put their heads together and came up with an excellent list of safe alternatives to chemical keyboard cleaners, including inexpensive keyboard vacuums that plug into your USB port, keyboard brushes and microfiber dusters, manual air blowers that look like turkey basters (Larry insisted on including a picture), and the ingenious method of turning your keyboard upside down to shake out debris.

Scotchgard, Teflon, Static Guard, Febreze, Magic Wrinkle Releaser (it's not bottled magic, I checked). . . . Do we really need any of these products? Are they worth the risk? You know what Shirli and Larry would say, and they can be very persuasive.*

A JABBERWOCK† AMONG US

Not to worry, we are finally getting around to the last major sources of fluoride you are likely to encounter in modern life as I know it. To bring the story full circle, we'll end this chapter with a discussion of other sources of fluoride forced upon us directly by uffish dentists.‡

---

*See what I mean? www.HiddenCauseofAcne.com/not-bottled-magic

†Jabberwock is derived from the anglo-saxon word *wocor,* meaning "offspring" or "fruit," combined with *jabber,* meaning "excited and voluble discussion." Therefore a jabberwock signifies "the result of much excited and voluble discussion." I find it a fitting title for this section.

‡For a description of unfamiliar words in this section, see https://en.wikipedia.org /wiki/Jabberwocky

We already talked about the fluoride that makes its way into our diet from the water supply, but how are we affected by the continual use of fluoridated water that fills our showers, sinks, bathtubs, hot tubs, swimming pools, steam rooms, humidifiers, dialysis machines, colonic machines, enema bags, fish tanks, koi ponds, and borogove baths? The dentists haven't gotten around to studying these avenues of fluoride exposure yet.

I'm happy to report that we can cross dialysis machines off our list of sources of fluoride exposure we need to worry about. Unfortunately, dialysis patients had to learn this lesson the hard way. I don't have any experience with dialysis machines, but from what Internet tells me, they were modified to filter out fluoride when doctors in the 1970s noticed dentists' infatuation with fluoride had condemned kidney patients to the accumulation of large amounts of fluoride in their bones and blood, leading to a bone disorder called osteomalacia.*

But what about the other means of fluoride exposure mentioned above? Even though we've been bathing our babies in fluoridated water for the last seventy years, I was not able to find any U.S. studies or statistics on the dermal absorption of the hydrofluorosilicic acid contained in the water supply. Reports of skin reactions from toothpaste and fluoridated steroid creams show that topical contact with fluoride can cause acne. The question is, at what concentration of fluoride are we affected? I will tell you my experience, but this is one of those questions that might require some investigative work on your part.

At the moment, my husband and I are temporarily living in an apartment outside Washington, D.C., where the water is fluoridated at 0.7 ppm. I am able to maintain clear skin even though I regularly shower and wash my hands in fluoridated water. However, when I first diagnosed my fluoroderma I lived in a condo fluoridated at 1 ppm, and my acne did not heal completely until I moved to a nonfluoridated neighborhood. Perhaps if I had stayed in Fluorideville long enough I

---

*You can read more about this at fluoridealert.org/issues/health/kidney

would have eventually been able to live there without my skin breaking out, but at the time it seemed like the amount of fluoride they added to the water was too much for my skin to handle, even though I was limiting my exposure as much as I knew how. Based on these past experiences, my current approach is to minimize my exposure to topical sources of fluoride when possible without being obsessive about it. I don't worry about water touching my face in the shower, but I don't intentionally rub it in either.

In my experience, fluoride exposure from the shower is the trickiest source to avoid. It is possible to filter fluoride from your shower, but it's not an easy fix because standard shower filters don't remove fluoride (for more information, see www.HiddenCauseofAcne.com/fluoride -filters). Since my primary residence in Florida is not fluoridated, my current approach is simply to not spend as much time in the shower anytime I suspect the water from the faucet might be fluoridated.

A study of fluoride and sodium lauryl sulfate (SLS), a chemical found in a variety of cleansers and shampoos, found that SLS increases fluoride absorption in the mouth by nine percent (Barkvoll 1990). Does it increase the absorption of fluoride through the skin too? I don't know and I don't know if anyone else knows either. It appears those studies have not been conducted.

Other avenues of topical fluoride exposure are much easier to avoid. You can wear gloves while doing the dishes, and it's only a small inconvenience to wash your face with bottled water instead of water from the faucet. When I lived in Newport, where they added particularly high amounts of fluoride, I remember washing my face with tap water and feeling a burning sensation on my skin. The experience convinced me to switch to using bottled water even though I knew nothing about fluoride at the time. I now wash my face with bottled water whenever I'm traveling.

Washing your face with bottled water isn't weird. The frabjous Cameron Diaz does it too. (Contrary to widespread reports in the media, she uses an assortment of brands, not just Evian. That would

be weird.) In her 2013 book, *The Body Book,* Cameron describes how she suffered from chronic acne even as an adult, just like I did. Pictures show it was concentrated around her mouth and chin, just like mine.*
Also like me, she tried all the popular treatments on the market—oral, topical, even the harshest prescriptions—but nothing worked for long.

At thirty years old, Cameron Diaz had a health awakening and started being conscious of the quality of the food she was eating. (Wait, am I Cameron Diaz?) She attributes her recovery from adult acne to the healthy home-cooked meals that replaced her fast-food addiction. Like Cordain's paleo dieters, Cameron explains her skin wasn't completely healed after she stopped eating fried jubjub nuggets, but it was significantly better. Whose wouldn't be? I don't doubt that her diet is greatly improved after ditching fast food, but I suspect the change in her acne was because she happened to eliminate significant sources of fluoride at the same time.†

While I tolerate showering and washing my hands in fluoridated water, baths are a different story. I haven't conducted any scientific studies on this, but to my little layman brain, it seems as if there would be a difference between standing in a shower where the water is obliged by gravity to constantly move toward the drain versus submerging your body for twenty minutes or more as if taunting the water to move inward.

In a study published in the *Journal of Public Health,* a research group led by Halina Brown, a toxicologist from the Massachusetts Department of Environmental Protection, analyzed the dermal absorp-

---

*To see what I mean, visit www.HiddenCauseofAcne.com/celebrities
†If anyone can convince Cameron to read this book, I will give both you and Cameron a free T-shirt of your choosing featuring any of the following popular themes: Shirli and Larry's Guide to Musical Chairs, the latest ad for fried jubjub nuggets, or a bedazzled artistic rendering of the Grapeleaf Skeletonizer. Same applies for Emma Stone and Katy Perry, who also struggle with adult acne and are equally frabjous. You'll get two T-shirts for Olivia Munn since she is already speaking out like a superhero about how avoiding fluoride cleared her acne (according to an undated interview with Noah Lehava for Coveteur, Munn learned about it from Google, but I don't know if she's heard about the book). Check out www.HiddenCauseofAcne.com/celebrities for the latest updates on celebrities who support the cause.

tion of various contaminants (not fluoride) and found that absorption through the skin accounted for 29 to 91 percent of the total amount consumed through a similar oral dose (Brown, Bishop, and Rowan 1984). Whoa there, Halina. That is a serious observation. The team concluded that "skin absorption of contaminants in drinking water has been underestimated and that ingestion may not constitute the sole or even primary route of exposure." Again, whoa.

If the CDC ever starts to wonder about the dermal absorption of the only chemical intentionally added to public water supplies because of its systemic effect on the human body, Brown's article provides some helpful tips for designing such a test. First, she points out that most researchers who conduct dermal studies of this nature tend to oversimplify matters (cough, *dentists*) by soaking their subjects' hands in a test solution and then measuring either the amount of the chemical excreted in their urine and breath, or the change in the chemical's concentration in the test solution. Furthermore, these studies typically involve adult male test subjects. I have not done any experiments to be sure of this, but it seems to me that baby-aged ballerina hands, for example, would absorb contaminants at a different rate than would manxome middle-aged man hands.

Speaking of scrotums, Brown explains that hands aren't the proper limb to be using for these experiments since the epidermis on the hands is a greater barrier to penetration than other parts of the body. Scrotums, on the other hand, are more permeable than hands, are available on most test subjects used for modern medical studies, and are easily submerged due to their dangling topography. As Brown and her coauthors explain, "Penetration through the scrotum, in fact, is estimated to be 100 percent, as compared to 8.6 percent for the forearm " (1984).

As cited in the study, other factors that affect the rate of dermal absorption include damage to the skin (such as sunburn, cuts, jock itch, etc.), a history of skin conditions that deplete the stratum corneum (such as eczema, psoriasis, crabs, etc.), previous exposure, nutrition, ratio of body fat, current hydration, chemical composition of the skin, temperature and pH of the solution, and also the lipophilicity, polarity, volatility, solubility, molecular weight, and carbon number of the chemical in question, as well as the presence of various other chemical compounds that act as accelerants or otherwise enhance permeability. Even if all these factors are accounted for, Brown and her colleagues point out that some chemical compounds are stored in the body for relatively long periods of time (cough, *fluoride*), meaning they might be absorbed through the skin and still not show up in breath or urine twenty-four hours later.

Once dentists have created a dermal study for fluoridated water keeping all these factors in mind, to really do their due diligence they will then need to conduct studies to account for greater rates of other routes of absorption, including aural (through the ears), nasal (up the nose), sublingual (under the tongue), buccal (inside of the cheeks), and orbital (through the eyes). Until all those studies are done for various age groups and ethnicities in both males and females, it's hard to estimate exactly how much fluoride seeps into our bodies at bath time. But seep it does.

In the early 1930s, while American dentists were daydreaming of ways to save the world by turning tap water into mouthwash, European researchers were experimenting with fluoride for other motivations. They noticed that fluoride inhibits thyroid function (an effect we covered in chapter 3), so they started studying the use of fluoride to treat patients with overactive thyroids.

Researchers in Austria, Germany, Italy, and France published research describing their experiments treating hyperthyroidism through fluoride therapy. I have not been able to find full texts of these studies and even the abstracts I've located aren't in English, but from what I can gather through Google Translate and other bits of information from Internet, some of the European researchers successfully lowered thyroid activity through the use of fluoridated *baths*.* In an interview on Joseph Mercola's website, one source claims the baths only needed to last for

---

*For example, see "Therapy of hyperthyroidism with halogens" by Gorlitzer von Mundy at https://www.ncbi.nlm.nih.gov/pubmed/12982497 or Wilhelm May's 1950 book (in German) entitled *Die Basedowsche Krankheit, Jod und Fluor.*

twenty minutes to have an effect with water fluoridated at 4 to 5 ppm (Jeff Greene 2012). This concentration is significantly higher than current levels in the United States, but some of us bathe for longer than twenty minutes, plus we've been bathing in, drinking, and eating fluoride since our baby ballerina years (or baby ballerino years, for the gents).

Based on the limited information available about dermal absorption of fluoridated water, here is my approach to full-body submergence situations. Being a health nut, I naturally love detox baths of all sorts, but I *never* take baths in fluoridated water. I'm sure you would probably survive a fluoridated bath now and then if you are lucky,* but for me it's not worth the additional exposure. I would not be able to enjoy it anyway, knowing what I know about fluoride.

Also, I rarely swim in pools or soak in hot tubs other than my own. At our house in Florida, we are fortunate to have a saltwater pool and hot tub in our backyard, a setup that is not uncommon amongst Floridians. I do swim in the ocean, however, and "gotcha" dentists might point out that ocean water contains fluoride (they're really up on their natural fluoride sources). But as I mentioned previously, seawater contains a different composition of fluoride than the smokestack variety they choose to add to the public water supply (*gotcha!*). It also contains a lot of other minerals not found in tap water, any of which could affect how fluoride is absorbed by living tissue. Swimming in the ocean does not have a negative effect on my skin.

To be clear, I have absolutely no idea how much fluoride is contained in your typical pool water or if it is absorbed into the body. This is just how I, as a person living with fluoroderma, choose to handle these situations based on the limited information at hand and my preexisting dislike of public pools and hot tubs.

If reading those last few paragraphs made your heart sink at the thought of losing precious "me time" in the home spa, I'm sorry. This

---

*;) The winky face is to indicate I am being facetious here in case dentists try to take this quote out of context. Do you think dentists get the meaning of winky face? Never mind. Of course they do. They probably use it all the time, as in: fluoride is safe and effective ;)

is clearly your dentist's fault. But since I hate seeing you this way, I will let you in on a secret. There is a fantastic alternative I am planning to suggest to you in the very next chapter. I will keep it a surprise for now, but if you're like me it will leave you shouting *Callooh! Callay!* from the highest branch of the nearest TumTum tree.

Before we get there, however, there are a last few tricks you should be aware of that the Cult of Dental Fluoride has been known to use to sneak their venerated element into your everyday life.

Like any large-scale religion, various sects have arisen tailored to the temperaments and habits of local practitioners. While the orthodox fluoride tradition developed in the United States elevates the role of dental clergy over the flock, emphasizing the water-into-mouthwash miracle, sects in other parts of the world have a more salt-of-the-earth interpretation of fluoride scripture. In one sect, individual practitioners are welcomed into a priesthood of all believers as they perform a little fluoride miracle with every sprinkle of the family salt shaker. The sect originated in Switzerland in 1955 when a Swiss gynecologist pioneered the addition of fluoride to table salt. It took several decades to catch on, as these things often do, but because of a historical monopoly on the salt trade in Swiss cantons (a local government structure—you knew bureaucrats had to be involved somehow), most of the salt produced in Switzerland is now fluoridated (Marthaler 2005).

The practice of adding fluoride to salt was replicated to a limited extent in neighboring countries in Europe. Usually it is limited to home salt shakers, enabling individuals to have the option to faithfully sprinkle pesticide directly on their food or not, as desired.

According to a 2006 article published by Franz Gotzfried in *Schweiz Monatsschr Zahnmed,** the following is a list of European coun-

---

*Translation: My Little Swiss Monster Named Zahnmed. As you can tell, *Schweiz Monatsschr Zahnmed* is a religious magazine used to discuss historical and theological aspects of salt fluoridation. Zahnmed is the name of their fluoride deity. Or, if you want to go with the literal translation of what the words actually mean, it would be *Swiss Monthly Dental Publication.*

tries where fluoride is added to salt, with the number in parentheses being the percent of household salt that is fluoridated in each country: Austria (6 percent), Czech Republic (15 percent), France (65 percent), Germany (67 percent), Slovakia (unknown), Spain (10 percent), and Switzerland (88 percent).

Belgium bans fluoridated salt because it is poison, while in the Netherlands it is only produced for export (Gotzfried 2006). Fluoride missionaries spread the sect to countries in Latin America and the Caribbean, especially Jamaica, Costa Rica, Colombia, Mexico, Peru, and Uruguay (Gillespie and Baez 2005). The sect is rare in Africa and Asia, although the World Health Organization sponsored a few programs in areas of Madagascar, Laos, and Vietnam (Petersen and Phantumvanit 2012).

A disparate sect of believers shun fluoridated water and salt altogether and instead cling to prophecy about a land overflowing with milk and fluoride. As of February 2017, the Alliance for a Cavity Free Future lists Bulgaria, Chile, China, Peru, Russia, Thailand, and the United Kingdom as countries where fluoride is occasionally added to milk (usually powdered frankenmilk) for distribution to school systems and food assistance programs aimed at defenseless children.

Lest we become caught up in the religious fervor and forget our fluoride facts, just because these programs exist in small enclaves around the world does not mean they are safe or effective. According to a Cochrane review of milk fluoridation programs, there is no quality evidence that fluoridated milk prevents dental caries and no information on the potential health hazards (Yeung, Chong, and Glenny 2015). A Cochrane review of fluoridated salt was proposed in 2009, in part by two WHO dentists, but was later withdrawn because it did not meet Cochrane's methodological standards (Marinho et al. 2016). (My investigator instincts tell me there's a story there, but I will leave it for someone else to tell.)

There is one last situation in which you will need to be on high guard against fluoride exposure. It's the most dangerous source referenced in this entire chapter, but you will likely encounter it only once or twice per year and in just one place: your dentist's chair.

Fluoride gel and other fluoridated dental treatments such as varnishes, rinses, polishes, and so forth, contribute not just to chronic fluoride toxicity but are also a primary source of *acute* fluoride toxicity. Fluoride gels were introduced in the 1960s without any clinical evidence of being safe or effective (Ekstrand 1987). Who needs evidence when you have faith?

It took dentists a couple of decades to notice that a dangerous portion of the *12,300 ppm* of fluoride contained in dental gel was finding its way into their patients' bloodstreams, causing spikes 100 times greater than normal levels and sometimes lasting up to fourteen hours following treatment (Ekstrand and Koch 1980). Even when it's not swallowed, fluoride's high acidity enhances its entry directly into the bloodstream from buccal and sublingual absorption (Whitford, Callan, and Wang 1982). This is why many people experience stomach pain, nausea, headaches, and vomiting shortly after their dentist gives them a free toothbrush and gallops off to poison another unsuspecting patient.

What's that you say? Your cousin's best friend's sister is a dental hygienist, and she says none of her patients ever threw up after a dental cleaning? Well, that evidence sounds anecdotal, so let's ask Internet about it to see what other anecdota we can find. Internet: kids vomiting fluoride. Go . . . That was easy. The first link I clicked on is a post at Mothering.com with the heart-wrenching subject line, "My Kids Were Poisoned Today—Who To Write To." There are several more examples in the comments section of her post too.* So, you can tell your cousin's best friend's sister that it looks like vomiting from dental cleanings is a real thing.

Death from dental cleanings is also a real thing. It doesn't happen

---

*For links to internet comments referenced in this chapter, visit www.HiddenCauseofAcne .com/clues

often, but at least one incident was reported by the *New York Times* on May 24, 1974, when a Brooklyn boy named William Kennerly died after swallowing a fluoride varnish the hygienist painted on his teeth (McFadden 1979). The hygienist was engrossed in conversation during the treatment, and when she handed him a cup of water afterward, she forgot to tell him he was supposed to use it to rinse and spit, not to drink. Being that it was his first visit to the dentist, three-year-old William did what any three-year-old child would do and drank the cup of water the health care professional handed him.

When William started sweating, vomiting, and complaining of headache and dizziness before leaving the doctor's office, his mother appealed to the dentist for help but was told not to worry because it was just a routine treatment. Unsatisfied with his answer, she immediately took her son to the ambulatory pediatric care unit nearby where they waited for over two hours to see a doctor. She thought William had fallen asleep in the waiting room, but he had actually slipped into a coma. He died a few hours later after being transported to a local hospital.*

Apparently dentists still aren't aware of the dangers of fluoridated gel because they have never studied them. In 2015, the Cochrane Oral Health Group reviewed the available research on the safety and effectiveness of fluoride gels for preventing tooth decay (Marinho et al. 2016). Of course they found that most of the evidence on fluoride's effectiveness was of low quality, moderate at best. But they also concluded, "There is little information on adverse effects or on acceptability of treatment. Future trials should include assessment of potential adverse effects."

Let me repeat their conclusion in more everyday terms. Even though fluoride gels have been used in American dental clinics for over *fifty years* on children who are literally vomiting in the car on the way

---

*In case you ever find yourself suffering from fluoride toxicity after a dental treatment, at the supreme court hearing that followed, a doctor testified that William's life might have been saved if the dentist had simply given him a glass of saltwater (although poison control experts doubt the efficacy of such a treatment and recommend intravenous calcium instead).

home, few studies have been carried out on their adverse health effects. Who needs studies when you have faith?

> *It was all very well to say "Drink me," but the wise little Alice was not going to do that in a hurry. "No, I'll look first," she said, "and see whether it's marked 'poison' or not"* . . . *she had never forgotten that if you drink much from a bottle marked "poison," it is almost certain to disagree with you, sooner or later. However, this bottle was not marked "poison," so Alice ventured to taste it, and finding it very nice, (it had, in fact, a sort of mixed flavour of cherry-tart, custard, pine-apple, roast turkey, toffee, and hot buttered toast,) she very soon finished it off.*
>
> LEWIS CARROLL,
> *ALICE'S ADVENTURES IN WONDERLAND*

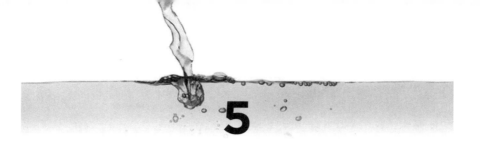

5

Healing Breakouts Overnight

Even miracles take a little time.

CINDERELLA'S FAIRY GODMOTHER

SKINCARE PRODUCTS ONLY PLAY a bit part in our story. If you develop your skill at avoiding the fluoride sources described in the previous chapter, you won't have to worry about breakouts anymore no matter what your skincare routine is. You will be one of those people who can sleep in makeup (or if you're like me, dog saliva) for three weeks straight without so much as a stressed pore. But there must be something that can be done to help the poor unfortunate souls who are in the midst of a fluoroderma flare-up.

Until you learn how to dust off all the traces of fluoride's fingerprints in your daily life, this chapter offers a little touch of magic to get you through any existing or future breakouts quickly, sometimes as fast as overnight. But first, a spell has been cast and we need to break it. Potent potions will emerge from competing cauldrons. And when we finally reach the start of our story, we will all be transformed from merfolk into humans.*

---

*If you aren't into skincare products (or musicals), feel free to skip the next section in this chapter and go directly to Oz, where a little mermaid (no, not *that* little mermaid) will help to elucidate exactly how fluoride causes acne.

A POISONED PART OF YOUR WORLD

The spells cast by the beauty industry are so powerful and pervasive that it is hard to find a modern woman who does not take a bite from its tampered fruit, sometimes partaking of the whole orchard before realizing who she is dealing with. We think we are presented with so many options when we browse the product aisles, but in reality most stores only offer one kind of skincare product: the dangerous kind. If you just don't see how a world that makes such wonderful things could be bad, let's flip through the pages of a typical beauty magazine together for a moment, shall we?

Look at this stuff. Isn't it sweet? Wouldn't you think our beauty cabinet's complete? Wouldn't you think we're the consumers who have everything? The visages are angelic, the scenery divine. Products cloaked in ruby packaging enchant the viewer's eye. A familiar face entices you to give the brand a try. But inside lurks a potion made of placental extract,* Teflon,† and a token butterfly.

Since that was so fun, now let's stroll arm in arm through a big box beauty store. *C'mon!*

Look at this store, treasures and more. How many marvels can one girl shop for? Looking around here you think, "Sure, they've got everything." And it's not just chemical products. They've got gizmos

---

*"Placental extracts, probably with high concentrations of the hormone progesterone and estrogenic chemicals, are sometimes used in cosmetics and hair care products, particularly products marketed to women of color. . . . Research indicates that use of these products in infants and children may also be linked to precocious puberty or early sexual maturation, a risk factor for later life breast cancer." See "Hormones in Personal Care Products" at https://www.bcpp.org/resource_topic/personal-care-products

†"Newly published test results show that a toxic contaminant linked to cancer known as perfluorooctanoic acid (PFOA) was found in anti-aging products from beloved brands Garnier and CoverGirl. PFOA is a contaminant of polytetrafluoroethylene (PTFE), an ingredient used to create a smooth finish on some cookware and personal care products." See "New Report from Breast Cancer Fund's Campaign for Safe Cosmetics Reveals Toxic Contaminants in L'Oréal Garnier and P&G Cover Girl Products" at http://www.safecosmetics.org/about-us/media/press-releases/chemical-linked-to-breast-cancer-found-in-popular-anti-aging-skin-care-products

and gadgets galore. You want whatzamahoos? They've got twenty, plus a selection of 200 more online. But who cares? It's not a good deal. We deserve *more*.

When I inhale the aroma from a newly opened jar of moisturizer, I want to feel like I'm right there where the flowers are. I want to see, want to smell them blossom. Breathing in all that, what do you call it? Oh—nature. Relying on synthetic chemicals, you don't get too far. Plants are required for distilling, extracting . . . infusing into a—what's that word again?—*nontoxic* personal care product.

The reason our beauty products are full of dangerous chemicals is because the entire $71 billion industry is regulated by a mere 591 words of legislation written into the Federal Food, Drug, and Cosmetic Act of 1938. Yes, it was *1938* when that happened.

Can you imagine your great-grandpa trying to write federal code to regulate the ingredients in your makeup bag? He tried his best to ensure it wouldn't contain substances that are "poisonous," "adulterated," or "putrid."* But Grandpa, poisonous is such a subjective term. What about carcinogenic, endocrine-disruptive, or lethal to unborn children? He didn't think of those. He also didn't think to require anyone to approve new products before they are put on the market, or to mandate that new chemicals be tested for health effects. Just in case that last line didn't hit you the way it should, I repeat it here in operatic falsetto: *no one is testing and approving our beauty products.*†

---

*You can read the current legislation in United States Code, Title 21, Chapter 9, Sub-chapter VI, sections 361–364 at http://uscode.house.gov/view.xhtml?path=/prelim@title21/chapter9/subchapter6&edition=prelim

†When the lack of regulation started to give the cosmetics industry a bad reputation, the industry itself set up a Cosmetics Ingredient Review panel to at least give the appearance of propriety. Out of over ten thousand unique chemicals used in personal care products, the industry panel has declared only eleven ingredients or chemical groups to be unsafe in its thirty-plus year history. Furthermore, companies are not required to avoid those chemicals in their products. So no, that does not count as regulation. See The Environmental Working Group, "Myths on cosmetics safety" at http://www.ewg.org/skindeep/myths-on-cosmetics-safety

All efforts to update federal regulation of cosmetics have been subverted by the personal care product industry. Did I mention they make $71 billion per year? When it comes to talk about safety, they don't like a lot of chatter. They think talking about toxins is a bore. In D.C. it's much preferred for shoppers not to say a word. After all dear, what are federal bureaucrats for? Come on, they're not all that impressed with scientific evidence. True partisans avoid it when they can. But they'll orate on and on about a scientist who's a pawn. Few chemicals that cause cancer have been banned. (*Cymbals!*)

To peddle their poison they, not coincidentally, know a bit of magic. It's a marketing talent they pay a lot of money to possess. And dear reader, let's be clear; they use it to stoke fear in the vulnerable, downtrodden, and distressed. Pathetic.

When your face is covered in breakouts, you'll take desperate measures to feel human again. I was once one of those poor, unfortunate souls. It's sad but true. We go flocking to their cauldrons crying, "Spells, Ulta, please!" And they help us. Or at least we think they do.

What other option do we have? Either we slather our faces in potentially toxic sludge or hide in our seashells all day. Life's full of tough choices, isn't it?

The solution to our problem is simple. The only way to get what you want is to become a cosmetics regulator yourself. "Can you do that?" My dear, sweet reader, that's what I do. That's what consumer advocacy groups like the Campaign for Safe Cosmetics and the Environmental Working Group live for—to help unfortunate consumers like ourselves. Poor souls with nowhere else to turn to. Online resources like SafeCosmetics.org and the Skin Deep Database* make it easy to research the potential health effects of the questionable concoctions included in your beauty balm.

But be forewarned. Reading labels doesn't always help. Some of the most noxious chemicals won't be listed on the bottle. Since none of the

---

*See www.ewg.org/skindeep

federal agencies are regulating personal care products, there is no one to require companies to put toxic or allergenic ingredients on product labels. Grandpa didn't think of that rule either. The system he set up to protect us from industry hazards is a complete failure. Sorry, Grandpa, but it's true.

We are smart young women, sick of swimming in a sea of questionable cosmetics. Ready to make a stand. Ready to know what the manufacturers know. Ask them our questions and get real answers. Like what's in this mascara and why does it, what's the word . . . *BURN!*

Oh, and there is one more thing. We haven't discussed the subject of payment. You can't buy something for nothing, you know. And I'm not just talking about the price tag. There's another small price they ask of you when you purchase a mass-marketed beauty product. It's a token really, a trifle. What they want from you is—your voice.

Every time you purchase a personal care product, you are voicing your support for the retailer, the manufacturer, and the entire regulatory system that enabled the product to be conjured into being. Now it's happened once or twice, someone had to pay an even bigger price, and I'm afraid coal tar is *still* not banned eighty-plus years later.* The beauty industry has had more than the odd complaint. On the whole they've *not* been saints to us poor unfortunate souls.

The long-term solution isn't just to purchase the "natural" line from the same old companies at the same old retail outlets. They might admit that in the past they've been nasty. (I wasn't kidding when I called them, well, a witch.) But they'll claim that nowadays they've mended all their ways. Repented, seen the light, and made a switch. True? No.

These companies are too big to care about individual tadpoles, even if they wanted to. They have portfolios to maintain, stockholders to appease, and decades of procedure to determine which direction they

---

*"In 1933, a woman was hospitalized with excruciating eye pain. Doctors watched in horror as her eyes were eaten away as though by acid. The culprit turned out to be an eyelash-darkening treatment called Lash Lure, which contained paraphenylenediamine, a toxic coal tar dye" (Sigurdson, 2013).

will swim. They might ride the currents of consumer trends and use their mystical marketing powers to take on the appearance of younger companies who genuinely build their brands on the use of pure and organic ingredients, but that does not disguise the fact that they are old outmoded corporations at heart. If you continue purchasing from them, you'll have red lips, your painted face, but don't underestimate the importance of *fine-print legal language.*

So go ahead. Make your choice. If you want to keep on buying the same cosmetics at Macy's, I understand.* You're a very busy woman and you haven't got all day to find a replacement for your favorite face cream. It won't cost a lot. Just your voice. If you want to use the turnpike then you've got to pay the toll. Take a last look at it now 'cause you're about to sell your soul. Johnson & Johnson, now they've got you, girls. The beauty industry's on a roll. You poor, unfortunate soul.

[Intermission]

While you would make a charming addition to the beauty industry's little garden of wayward spirits, you don't need a kiss from a prince, your adopted stepmother, or even your sister to wake up from their spell. If I know you, the waves of doubt are already rising to the forefront of your mind. Maybe a Brazilian blowout gave you hypotrichosis (Greek caveman for "depressed hair condition," or hair loss), and now you are questioning the concoctions of shampoo on your shower shelf (Sigurdson and Roth 2015). Maybe you are wondering about your monthly manicure after reading the *New York Times* article about the high incidence of salon workers who have lung diseases, miscarriages, and special-needs children because of their work in the industry (Maslin Nir 2015).

You might not know why, but you're dying to try—you want to kiss

---

*The Campaign for Safe Cosmetics ranked Macy's at the bottom of the list of retailers who support the use of safe cosmetics. Macy's does not have a policy to screen for personal care products of concern. Instead, the company has stated that current regulatory standards are adequate for ensuring personal care product safety. Macy's relies on vendors to meet safety standards (Campaign for Safe Cosmetics 2012).

goodbye to conventional beauty products. Well, now's your moment, floating in a blue lagoon of fluorescent chemical fabrications. Girl, you better do it soon. No time will be better.

It might appear as if the big commercial beauty corporations are the rulers of the ocean, but you have other options. You won't find them at most national retail chains, but some companies stake their reputations on the integrity of their wizardry. Handcrafted, wild harvested, infused with good intentions—these are the kinds of ingredients you will find on their labels. Some retailers too, like Whole Foods Market, set their own standards about what chemicals they allow in their cupboards.*

In 2004, a nonprofit group sponsored the Compact for Safe Cosmetics asking manufacturers to sign a pledge to fully disclose ingredients, to avoid the use of chemicals banned in other countries, and to prohibit the use of those linked to cancer or birth defects. By 2011, the campaign listed over 500 manufacturers who satisfied their standards for healthier products.

Zut alors, they have missed one! *Sacre bleu,* what is this? How on earth could they miss such a sweet little succulent beauty product manufacturer. I'm referring to *you.* Homemade beauty products and single-ingredient potions are some of the most luxurious beauty treatments in the world. Since I am a simple kind of merwoman, this is the option I often use for myself. For example, diluted raw apple cider vinegar makes for a refreshing toner. And for a moisturizer—some coconut oil, just a dab.† Homemade beauty treatments are an essential part of the everyday health tradition in many cultures, from the *mandi bunga* flower baths of Malaysia to the famous scented ayurveda oils of India. *Quel domage,* what a loss that we forgot how to make our own sauce.

But not all of us have forgotten, or if we did, we are now starting to remember. Relying on little more than their kitchen sinks, kitchen counters, and kitchen gardens, a new cadre of modern sorceresses has

*Whole Foods Market ranked #1 on the Campaign for Safe Cosmetic's list of retailers who support the use of safe personal care products (Campaign for Safe Cosmetics 2012).
†For more information on the products I use, see www.HiddenCauseofAcne.com/skincare

taken root throughout the country as they experiment with the lost art of beauty alchemy. I met one such phoenix online during my blogging years. Maggie's degree is in architecture from Harvard's Graduate School of Design, but now she works as a mixer of potions, evoking the scents of her native Persia from her West Hollywood kitchen. Her company, Lalun Naturals, is named after a village in the Alborz Mountains of Iran where she picnicked under a walnut tree with her family as a child.

Ordering a potion from Maggie is like having your own personalized apothecary. A magical one, of course. She sells a skincare line that changes with the seasons—lavender in summer, calendula in fall, rosehips in winter, and orange blossoms in spring. Maggie's creations are so exclusive they aren't sold in stores, but they are readily available to those who seek them on her website and on Etsy.*

In fact, Etsy is filled with personal care products from magicians like Maggie. Reminiscing just now about the scent of her inspired winter rose moisturizer made from rosehip seed, raw shea butter, and macadamia oil, I had a vision of what the world would look like if more people knew they could buy exquisite personal care products from micro-companies like Maggie's. That world has fewer synthetic chemicals, fewer side effects. More gardens, more Maggies. Instead of waiting to start gardening in retirement, more people are able to follow their natural passion for plants and flowers, working out of their homes creating herbal works of art.

Internet proposes that artists like Maggie don't need their creations to go viral to be successful. It is possible they could make a healthy living with a modest number of devotees.† The story of industrialization (and Cinderella) would lead us to believe that companies that start in basements need to end up in corporate castles to be considered a success. But what if instead of going to the ball, Cinderella stayed home and

---

*www.lalunnaturals.etsy.com
†See "1,000 True Fans," by Kevin Kelly at kk.org/thetechnium/1000-true-fans

read *The 4-Hour Workweek* by Tim Ferris (2007) and then set up her own small business selling natural cleansers, lotions, and other beauty products online? Might she have freed herself from her evil stepmother and lived out her days singing show tunes to adoring forest creatures while foraging for wild herbs with Jaq and Gus-Gus? (They would have been so good at that.) Who knows, maybe her happily ever after would have been even happier.

Looking around at our present situation, I know it will take more than a few chants of "bibbidy-bobbidy-boo" to transform the beauty industry into an independent network of fairy godmothers.* But we buy in to the current model with every lotion we purchase. What if we bought into the fairy-tale model instead?

What would I give to live in a world without triclosan? What would I pay to keep you away from BHA? What would I do just to see you smiling at me with lead-free lipstick? Carcinogen-free, wish we could be part of that world.

When's it our turn? Wouldn't I love not to gauge our beauty products by what they're free of . . .

[Finale]

Now that we know acne-free skin does not require the use of special skincare products, our facial potions—like all fine works of art—are free to exist purely for the pleasure that comes with indulging our senses in the sweet scents and textures of the natural world, with the added bonus of providing a little extra luminescence when desired.

A better beauty industry already exists; we don't need to wait for government princes to take us there. The alchemists who create such masterpieces are already among us, we just need to find and support them until we reach the tipping point and their good magic spreads throughout the land. I know it won't happen overnight, but if you believe in fairy-tale endings, I will believe in them too. Now, do we have a deal?

---

*Why do I picture them all flying around in pink Cadillacs?

If you haven't done so already, you can start to build this new world by choosing just one type of personal care product in your repertoire and finding a version that supports our shared vision for what the beauty industry should look like.* It doesn't have to be a Maggie. Just find a source that defines itself on the use of nothing but quality ingredients, and then try to purchase it through a retailer who takes care not to poison masses of people with their products.

The key is not to put it off. Choose a product from your bathroom shelf *right now*. We mustn't lurk in doorways, it's rude.

[Reprise]

I don't know when. I don't know how. But I know something's starting right now. Watch and you'll see. Someday we'll be part of *that* world.

A MERMAID VISITS OZ

To understand which skincare treatments are the most effective at healing breakouts, we need to revisit an unanswered question that arose in part 1 of our story. What exactly is going on inside our bodies that causes the fluoride we eat and drink to end up on our faces? I have a theory, but it requires us to try to view the human body with fresh eyes. Here is a story designed to help us do just that.

In *The Little Mermaid* when Ariel has a question about "human stuff," she ventures to the surface to ask her seagull friend, Scuttle. Let's say for the purpose of this exercise that one day, a similar mermaid who is not a copyrighted Disney character—let's call her Aquaria—starts wondering about the physiology of humans that allows them to live outside of the water. (If you must know, yes, Aquaria is in love with a human and is trying to figure out how they could be together. It happens.) She decides to visit the favorite resting spot of her pelican friend,

---

*For some suggestions to get you started, see www.HiddenCauseofAcne.com/skincare

Gully, to see if he can provide any information on how a human and a mermaid might be able to make things work.

When Aquaria arrives at Gully's place, he just so happens to be having lunch with America's favorite doctor, Mehmet Oz. It doesn't take long before Aquaria is interrogating Oz about human physiology. The good doc doesn't seem to mind and quickly whips out an autographed copy of his bestselling book, *You: The Owner's Manual.* Flipping to the table of contents, he explains that each chapter covers a major system of the human body. You've got the heart and veins, the brain, the musculoskeletal system, the lungs, the gut, the sexual organs, the sensory organs, the immune system, and finally, the hormonal system.

Aquaria tries to listen politely but she can't keep her mind from wandering back to her mermaid anatomy class in high school. Mermaids have hearts and brains and muscles and bones. Like their friendly neighbors, the dolphins, they even have lungs. But why is it that if she tried to live with humans on land she would shrivel and die like a beached whale?

Aquaria interrupts the doc just as he was getting to the good part about homocysteine and arterial inflammation. "But how do they live outside the ocean?!" she demands.

Sensing his aquatic guest was losing her patience, Gully jumps in with an explanation. "Out of the ocean? Oh, yes. Excellent question." He clears his throat, "In prehysterical times when humans first decided to live out of the ocean, they just took the ocean with 'em." He then grabs Dr. Oz by both ears and stares deeply at his forehead. "Yep, there it is," he states as a matter of fact. "I can see it leaking out of his big water-balloon skull right now."

Gully motions for Aquaria to view the drops of moisture percolating on Oz's brow. "You see?" he says triumphantly. "Saltwater."

Not wanting to be shown up by a know-it-all pelican, Dr. Oz tries to recompose himself by resorting to an old doctor's tactic (you probably saw this one before) where he throws out a statistic to demonstrate his expertise on a topic. "Actually, Gully is on to something here," Dr. Oz says as he runs his hands through his hair in an attempt to reshape it back into an aesthetically pleasing configuration. "About two-thirds of the human body is water."

Aquaria raises an eyebrow in suspicion. "If the human body is mostly water, then why isn't *water* one of the chapters in your book?" she asks. Dr. Oz stops to think for a moment.

"In fact," she continues, "if the human body is mostly water, shouldn't it be the very first chapter?" With Oz at a loss for words, Aquaria instinctively turns to chapter 1 in search of an answer to her own question.

"Look!" she shouts, pointing emphatically. "Right here on page 3 you say: 'your heart is your water main.' How poetic!" Aquaria sighs and hugs the book to her chest before asking, "In the human body, is the heart pumping water?"

Dr. Oz shakes his head. This is not going at all like the conversations he has with human women on television. "That was just an analogy," he explains. "The heart pumps *blood* through the body, providing nutrients for all the organs and tissues. It's the most life-giving organ we have, which is why I wrote about it first. It's why people write poems about it and use its image to decorate candy boxes, boxer shorts, and Valentine's Day cards."

A deflated Aquaria flips through a few more pages, but her mind starts to wander. When she looks up, Gully's guest is waxing poetic about aortic valves. He was just making his way back to the good part about homocysteine when she thinks up an excuse about missing a concert for her father and swims off into the fathoms below.

By submerging us in Aquaria's point of view with this silly story, my hope is that it will help you see the human body at least a little differently. We tend to fixate so intensely on our modern interpretations that we forget they are only a story of the world, not the world itself. Despite Dr. Oz's admirable intention to write a book that explains all the major parts of human anatomy in everyday terms, he and his coauthor, Dr. Michael Roizen, chose not to include a chapter on the body's extensive saltwater circulatory system.

Did you know your body has an extensive saltwater circulatory system? I wouldn't blame you if you didn't since it has been historically neglected in Western medicine. It is called the lymphatic system, and if my theory is correct, it is integral to understanding the mystery of how fluoride causes acne.

The lymphatic system is comprised of a network of vessels that circulate a clear fluid called lymph, a term that comes from the Latin word *lympha,* meaning "water." Like sweat and tears, lymph is basically a type of saltwater. It originates as plasma, the yellow liquid component of blood. The lymphatic system has long been overshadowed by the more colorful blood circulatory system because it doesn't have a flamboyant character like the heart to help circulate lymph around the body. We tend to focus on organs we can hold in our hands or feel beating under our chest, but lymph vessels are difficult to observe even upon dissection. The lymphatic system wasn't even discovered in Western medicine until the seventeenth century when some guys in Sweden and Denmark who no one cares about anymore anyway started fighting over who noticed it first.

The human body contains twice as much lymph as it does blood, which makes Aquaria wonder why Oz went *on and on* about the cardiovascular system but didn't think to tell her about the liters of saltwater circulating through his body at that very moment. In his book, he mentions the lymphatic system as a brief side note in the chapter on immunity, right below his description of the thymus, bone marrow, and spleen (a. k. a. the super-boring parts no one cares about unless they have to). He doesn't think to acknowledge the existence of lymph or the extensive system of lymphatic vessels that extend to every organ and tissue in the body. Dr. Oz describes the lymphatic system a little differently on his blog where he compares it to the drainpipes on a house that lead to the sewer. In the land of Oz, the heart is the body's water main while lymph is dirty toilet water. We can tell stories about nature, but our stories will never capture its full being.

It is true that one of the purposes of the lymphatic system is to transport metabolic waste away from the cells. Lymph can contain a variety of substances, including lipids, proteins, enzymes, hormones, urea, dissolved gases, bacteria, viruses, and other cellular debris. Lymph also plays an important role in the immune system by transporting white blood cells, also known as lymphocytes, to and from lymph nodes that act as filters that rid the body of toxic substances. When doctors check along the sides of a patient's neck for swollen glands, they are feeling to see if the lymph nodes are enlarged and thereby fighting an infection.

The lymphatic system might play a small supporting role in Western views of the human body, but it is a central concept in Eastern medicine where for centuries the idea of lymph was bound up in conceptions of *qi* or *prana,* or it was expressed simply as "damp." The term *lymph* is limited to fluid that is contained inside lymphatic vessels, but before this fluid enters the lymphatic vessels, it is considered interstitial fluid—the fluid that bathes our cells. Therefore, the defining characteristic that differentiates interstitial fluid from lymphatic fluid is location. But regardless of where it is located in the body, isn't it all just saltwater? Dr. Oz might think of lymph as dirty toilet water, but perhaps an inquisitive mermaid would find it more akin to the ever-present experience of *ocean.**

Now that Aquaria's line of inquiry has revealed the inner ocean that bathes every cell in the human body, we can more easily see how the fluoride we consume through our diet ends up on our faces the way a plastic bag on the beach ends up in the blowhole of a whale.

Immunity and detoxification are the two best-known roles for the lymphatic system, but lymph also plays an important part in digestion, specifically the digestion of fats. The average person is born with six to

*And then she would sing a lively song about it with a Rastafarian hermit crab who I did not include in this story because we had limited time for character development. However, if you listen attentively through the remainder of this chapter, at the end I promise to share with you the song they sing together. It is very catchy.

seven hundred lymph nodes distributed throughout the body, with more than half located in the abdominal region. The small intestine contains special lymphatic vessels called lacteals that absorb fat-soluble nutrients consumed in the diet. Water-soluble nutrients are passed directly to the liver for filtering, but fat-soluble nutrients like fluoride are taken up by the lymphatic system where they are transported to systemic circulation before making their way back to the liver via the bloodstream.

We like to define various bodies of water by their differences and give them each a name, but they are all part of the same ocean. That is why when you consume too much fluoride in your diet, your sweat smells different, your breath stinks, your tongue might turn white, and your skin desperately attempts to bail itself out by jettisoning the offending fluid overboard out the nearest pore. The pores in your skin act as a secondary egress route when the regular flow of lymph is congested. Approximately 70 percent of lymphatic flow takes place in the superficial lymph capillaries located just beneath the surface of the skin (Chikly 2001). If you pay close attention to the pattern of your breakouts, you might even be able to trace some of the pathways of the lymphatic vessels that drain lymph toward your heart.

When the waters of your inner ocean start to stagnate from over-pollution, there are many steps you can take to help them flow freely again. Now that you know my theory that fluoride causes acne by congesting your lymphatic system, it should be clear that any activity that improves lymphatic circulation will help to prevent and heal breakouts. Lymph circulates through a series of one-way valves that give the lymphatic system the characteristic appearance of a string of pearls (known in scientific parlance as "moniliform" shape). Without a pump, the lymphatic system relies on a type of peristalsis stimulated by a combination of skeletal movement and pressure changes in the chest cavity during breathing. In other words, lymph flows as a function of movement and breath.

For many Americans, there are two kinds of exercise: weight training and cardio. Notice they both focus on working your muscles. If your heart muscle is pounding at the recommended beat per minute, then you are maximizing your workout. But if we designed our exercises with the lymphatic system in mind, they would look a lot different. Instead of focusing exclusively on muscles, we would focus on stimulating lymphatic flow by leveraging movement with breath. We would probably move into certain positions we don't commonly use in daily life, and then take a deep breath to encourage that angle of lymphatic circulation. If we really wanted to shake lymph up, we would incorporate some movements that reverse the regular pull of gravity—you know, turn the lava lamp upside down and let the bubbles float to the top for a minute or two. To be acutely aware of our inner waterworld, we would spend centuries carefully observing the effects of breath on various poses, perhaps even developing complex breathing exercises to influence the tides and currents of the ocean within.

The lymphatic system is widely neglected in conventional approaches to health in the United States, but it's a different story in other parts of the world. While Americans focus on working their muscles, the exercise traditions in Asia are centered on movement and breath. Practices like yoga, tai chi, and qigong are ideal for improving lymphatic flow and consequently, the health of your skin.

In Europe, the lymphatic system is addressed through manual techniques where the skin is manipulated in a form of massage designed to enhance the circulation of lymphatic fluid. The most popular technique was developed by Emil and Estrid Vodder, two Danish physicians working in the south of France in the 1930s. It is now commonly used in European hospitals where it is prescribed by physicians and even reimbursed by insurance. Acne was one of the conditions the Vodders first treated with their lymph drainage technique. As I mentioned in chapter 1, I experienced relief from my cystic acne after a single session of a similar lymph drainage therapy developed by Dr. Chikly.

Yoga and massage might not be your typical skincare treatments, but I hope it is now apparent why they are more effective at healing acne than virtually any product you will find at . . .

Oh no. Stop everything. Was that a flash of disappointment I saw in your eyes just now? Don't tell me you're disappointed. I can't take it. You want to slather scented stuff on your face, don't you. You want to glob it on, rub it in, and soak in it like Miss Piggy in a fancy French mud bath. You want to put product on your skin *right now* to fix those appalling, painful pustules on your otherwise pretty face.*

Well, my friend, you don't think I would let you sink away discontented, did you? Now that you mention it, there are a few rituals you can perform in front of your bathroom mirror to banish existing breakouts on this very night. But be forewarned, you might need to gather some courage to attempt them. . . Mirror, mirror, on the wall, who's the bravest of us all?

> *You are not a drop in the ocean.*
> *You are the entire ocean in a drop.*
> RUMI

FROM BEAUTY TO
THE BEAST AND BACK

It's a tale as old as time. Humanity spends millennia painstakingly uncovering a hidden treasure of the natural world, then industrialization steps in and mutates it to the point doctors convince us we don't want it anymore and should do drugs instead.

While modern chemists frantically stir their cauldrons looking for the latest/greatest chemical ingredients to include in their so-called beauty products, the most effective skincare products were discovered ages ago. Some of them we've forgotten, but others have been vilified to the point you might cringe in fear at their very suggestion. But fear not. We already know how the story ends. (Spoiler alert: the Beast is Prince Charming in disguise.)

---

*Shut up. You're pretty.

Though few of us realize it, the most effective skincare product for acne is as plain as the nose on your face. Or to be more precise, it is as plain as the *oil* on the nose on your face. Thousands of years before soap came into widespread usage, people cleansed their skin with oil.

When your inflamed skin is already shining with "excess" oil, it might feel scary to put more oil on your face, but that's your dermatologist's story—the one where your acne-prone skin is caused by your crazy hormones and your overproductive oil glands. In our story, your acne-prone skin is caused by your crazy dentist and your overpolluted lymphatic system. Oil is the body's way of handling that congestion by sending extra fluid out through the pores. Cleansing your face with oil augments this natural process by helping dissolve fat-soluble substances on your skin.

Dermatologists might have succeeded in convincing us that cleansing oily skin with oil is a ludicrous idea, but chemists, nature, ancient Romans, and popular health bloggers like Mommypotamus tell us otherwise. In chemistry, the term lipophilicity is Greek caveman for "lipid loving." It refers to the ability of a chemical compound to dissolve in fats and oils. Over the years, chemists noticed that lipid-loving substances tend to dissolve in other lipid-loving substances. It is an axiom referred to as "like dissolves like." Water-loving (i.e., *hydro*philic) substances dissolve in other water-loving substances, but to dissolve the oil on your face, you will need another oil. This axiom of lipophilicity explains why bathers in the famous baths of ancient Rome cleansed their skin by rubbing oil into their bodies and then scraping it off using a curved metal tool called a *strigil*.

Traditional oils like olive and coconut have a long history of use for skincare in many cultures. But if oil is so great at cleansing oily skin, then why does it have such a bad reputation for clogging pores? That's a good story. How about we let Matthew McConaughey tell it.

After growing up in nonfluoridated Uvalde, Texas, Matthew moved to fluoridated Longview, Texas, prior to high school where he developed a severe case of acne. His mom was selling cosmetics door-to-door and suggested he try a product she was peddling, oil of mink. (To say it like Matthew, you need some extra drawl on the word *oil*. Like this: "ooooooil of mink." Good.)

McConaughey tells the rest of the story to Jimmy Fallon on *The Tonight Show*, "So I start doing the mink oil masks at night, and my face is starting to swell up, and I'm developing really bad acne. I talked to my dad's secretary, who turned my mom on to it. I'm really concerned. And the lady's like, 'Wow, you just sure have a lot of impurities, Matthew. Keep it up! And we'll just pull all of the impurities out, and you'll never have a blemish again.'"

The story ends with Matthew visiting the dermatologist, who predictably chides him to stop putting oil on his already oily face and instead gives him a bottle of Inflammatory Bowel Disease (i.e., acne medication). His mother sues the manufacturer of her mink oil product for $30,000 but loses when the judge is shown a photograph that proves Matthew was still voted Most Handsome in his high school class.

Looking at Matthew McConaughey's acne story, it is not that different from the tale dentists tell about fluoridation. His mom, his dad's secretary, and teenaged Matthew himself are the helpless and confused townspeople. The dermatologist is the wise hero. Industrial poison is the magic potion the hero uses to save the day. The judge is the government official who sides with industry lawyers because of a distracting but irrelevant picture of a smiling child with sparkly white teeth.

If we didn't know better, stories like Matthew's seem to confirm the idea that oil causes acne. But just like in the story of fluoridation, an industry chemist and a few admen are trying their best to hide behind a cardboard cactus on the back of the stage.

What is this mysterious "oil of mink" the big bad beauty industry was marketing to women and our future leading men in the 1980s? We find some insight to this question in a document written in 1994 (thank you, Internet) by DeeVon Bailey and Michael Thomsen at the University of Utah in which they outline their diabolical plot for Utah to take over the mink oil manufacturing world. Or at least the coveted *cosmetics* mink oil manufacturing world. Or maybe just the leather care market. Or perhaps they could sell it to local shoe stores? Or they could create their own shoe stores and then sell it to them? Anyway.

The document explains that most mink oil in Utah is marketed as a low-grade oil used primarily to feed factory-farmed livestock. Bailey's plot suggests that if Utah manufacturers adopted a fractional distillation process like those savvy mink companies in Wisconsin, then Utah mink oil might live a life of luxury in high-end beauty lotions or leather coats instead of ending up as cow caca. Bailey and Thomsen (1994) cite Avon and Kiwi as two companies that use "highly processed" mink oil in their product lines. They explain that cosmetics companies use mink oil in skincare products like creams and lotions, while leather care companies use it to treat, preserve, and waterproof leather.

Now, I'm not a beauty product manufacturer *or* a leather specialist, so I am doubly forced to rely on my little layman brain for this one, but if a product is able to keep fluids out, might it also have the effect of keeping fluids in? Even when those fluids are bodily fluids that aren't supposed to stay in? It makes sense why Mother Nature would use a waterproofing oil for a semiaquatic animal like mink, but as Matthew McConaughey selflessly tried to show us, waterproofing a human face might not be the best option for healing acne.

Ooooil of mink might sound luxurious, especially the way Matthew McConaughey says it, but it is not a traditional oil for skincare. As Dr. Bailey and his minions demonstrate, the use of mink oil in cosmetics is more an attempt by the fur industry to increase revenue by selling a by-product of imprisoned minks as something other than cheap fodder for imprisoned cows.

Dermatologists fail to differentiate this type of heavily processed industrialized oil from more traditional oils used for skincare when deciphering oil's role in the causes and cures for acne. While adolescent Matthew was slathering his future Oscar-winning face with mutated mink oil in the 1980s, people started noticing similar side effects from other industrialized cosmetic oils. In an attempt to throw consumers off their trail, industry marketers created a secret beauty product language consisting of words like *hypoallergenic, noncomedogenic,* and *dermatologist-approved*. Consumers assumed these new words meant someone was looking out for the safety of their beauty products and that potions inscribed with such symbols would not clog pores. But in legal terms, these are nonsense words, the way "chihuahua" is the color of pink lipstick.

Because of the mass confusion over the role of oil in the cause of acne, it was widely banished as a modern skincare cleanser in the latter half of the twentieth century. It remained locked away in a castle tower until Internet revived interest in it with a mysterious little website called TheOilCleansingMethod.com.

The site was created by Stephanie Strauss, a stay-at-home mom who in the early 1990s read a book that recommended cleansing your face with olive oil. The idea intrigued her, so she tried it and immediately fell in love with the soft, supple skin that resulted. She was also intrigued by a new toy called the World Wide Web and created a simple website to tell people about cleansing with oil. It was just a few pages, but after fifteen years online it managed to attract the attention of some of the most popular natural health and beauty bloggers, such as Mommypotamus, Crunchy Betty, and Wellness Mama.

Just like thousands of other American women in her demographic, Stephanie has adult acne and is prone to breakouts along her chin and jawline. She suggests using a castor oil blend to cleanse your face, but she also recommends mineral oil and the occasional light soaping with Johnson & Johnson's baby wash—two highly industrialized chemical products that show she has not yet fully awoken from the industry's spell.

You don't need to use a particular blend to cleanse your skin with oil. Castor oil is widely recommended because of Stephanie's site, but it is a potent medicinal oil that can cause strong reactions—it is made from the same plant used to produce ricin. Traditional skincare oils are nourishing in different ways, so you might have to experiment with a few oils to find the ones you like best. Jojoba, coconut, olive, and almond oil are some of the most versatile. Or you could consult a beauty mystic like Maggie who formulates her oil cleansers to balance with the seasons—extra hydrating in winter and more absorbent in summer months.

The way oils are grown and processed can also influence how they affect your face. Maggie only uses organic oils that are extracted using traditional cold-pressed methods. If your skin does not react well to a certain oil, remember the hard-earned lesson we learned from Matthew McConaughey: stop using it and try something else.

You don't need detailed instructions for oil cleansing either. The premise is simple. Massage a traditional oil used in skincare into your skin (as opposed to a highly processed industrialized oil used in mink enslavement, *Matthew!*). Then gently remove it. You can start with wet skin or dry skin. You can use circular motions or upward strokes. You can massage for thirty seconds or two minutes. You can remove the oil with a warm washcloth, a cold washcloth, a tissue, a cotton round, a potholder, a Matthew McConaughey T-shirt, a doily, or your dog's tongue. (Just kidding, I don't do that last one. Seriously, I don't.)

My favorite method for removing oil from my skin is a strigil-like tool similar to what the ancient Romans commonly used to scrape off oil and dead skin cells. I found it at a discount store several years ago. It was originally sold by QVC but is no longer on the market. A company created a similar product called LeEdge, but that seems to be out of production now too, replaced by a new product that I have not yet tried called Exfolimate. Clearly the market for Roman strigils is experiencing a moment of volatility, but I will try to keep you updated with the latest options at www.HiddenCauseofAcne.com/skincare.*

While strigil-like tools are the best facial exfoliators I know of, their utility is limited if you have active breakouts because they can only be

---

*Update: Instead of a strigil-like tool, I recently started exfoliating my skin with a facial cleansing brush from Clarisonic. So far, so good!

used on smooth skin. But there is another tool that has a longstanding tradition of use in conjunction with oils, and it is even more effective at improving lymphatic circulation.

Next to acupuncture, cupping therapy is the primary technique used in traditional Chinese medicine to reduce stagnation in qi and internal fluids. It was also practiced by early Egyptians before it spread to ancient Greece and many countries in Europe and even the Americas. In cupping therapy, cups are used to create suction against the skin, pulling the tissue upward like an inverse massage. The earliest references to cupping involved the use of animal horns and then jars made of bamboo or pottery. Glass cups eventually came into widespread use, but now silicone cups are readily available and make it easy to incorporate this ancient practice into your home skincare routine.

A gentle type of cupping called "glide cupping" is the treatment I relied on when I needed to heal a breakout quickly. I found it can even prevent a blemish from surfacing if I treat it early enough. Instructions for glide cupping are simple. After massaging your face with oil, squeeze the cup to create a light suction and then release it against your skin. Lymph capillaries are sensitive, so you only need to use enough suction to keep the cup attached. Then glide the cup across your face. You don't need to run the cup directly over the breakout for cupping to be effective. Doing so could aggravate already tender skin. Instead, focus on improving the overall flow of lymph. I like to start at my neck with several downward strokes before moving to the problem area on my chin and around the sides of my mouth. I'll also incorporate some long strokes along my jawline toward my ears and from the inside edge of my eyebrow across my forehead. The idea is to move in the general direction of lymphatic flow.*

In Stephanie's oil cleansing method, she recommends draping a hot towel over your face, "essentially steaming [y]our skin as an aesthetician

---

*For a video demonstration and more information on cupping to heal acne, visit www.HiddenCauseofAcne.com/facial-cupping

would, but without the luxury of a steam machine." A hot towel feels nice, but you also could have the luxury of a steam machine for about the same price as the Egyptian cotton washcloths Stephanie recommends on her site. Small facial saunas start at as little as twenty dollars and can work your skin into a healthy sweat in less than ten minutes. I found them to be much more effective than leaning over a bowl of hot water. Steaming your face won't prevent acne if you are still consuming fluoride, but it is an excellent treatment for those occasions when you accidentally consume some fluoridated California wine out of a dancing punchbowl, for example, and have a few breakouts you want to heal before an important date with a bewitched prince.

Depending on your powers of perception, you might have noticed at some point over the years that the skin on your face is connected to the rest of your body. While facial saunas are a great option if you are tight on money or space, they can't compare to the health benefits of a full body version. Saunas are a time-tested way to improve lymphatic circulation and therefore help maintain clear skin. From the sweat lodges of Mesoamerica to the weekly sauna rituals in northern Europe and the hammams of the Muslim world, saunas are a longstanding tradition in many cultures for improving skin health and general detoxification. It is a shame they have been largely abandoned in modern American life.

I did my part to bring back saunas after reading *Sauna Therapy for Detoxification and Healing* by Lawrence Wilson. At first, I used a far-infrared sauna purchased from a friend when she moved overseas. But eventually, I upgraded to a near-infrared sauna like Dr. Wilson recommends in his book. Near-infrared saunas are about the price of a MacBook, or you can build one yourself for under two hundred dollars. If you live in a fluoridated house and don't want to take baths in industrial pollution, they are the perfect alternative for thirty minutes of luxury "me time."

Let's see. We talked about cleansing your face with oil. We talked about increasing sweat. What other traditional skincare solutions have been neglected in recent years? Oh right, dirt.

One of the most effective remedies for healing breakouts quickly is dirt, or more specifically, clay. The first recorded use of medicinal clay was in ancient Mesopotamia, but some scholars (and Wikipedia) believe clay was used to heal wounds even in prehistoric times. Ancient Egyptians, Classical Romans, Medieval Persians, Renaissance Europeans, and Crunchy Californians all used clay as a traditional healing compound.

The term *bentonite* refers to a variety of absorbent clays derived from volcanic ash. There are a lot of scientific explanations for why bentonite clay is helpful in healing acne, but I didn't read any of them when I first started using it. I based my decision solely on the 6,000-plus reviewers who rave about bentonite clay on Amazon. A one-pound canister costs less than eight dollars.*

You can get super fancy with clay, but I followed the directions on the label and mixed a spoonful with equal parts organic apple cider vinegar and water. It whips into a delightful green froth that feels like marshmallow cream when first applied, but soon hardens your face into Venus de Milo. After just twenty minutes, my breakouts were well on their way to being ancient history. It was magic.

. . . Or science. Same diff. Bentonite clay is scientifically proven to be exceedingly good at absorbing human sebum. In fact, when scientists conduct studies on how much sebum is secreted by humans, they sometimes use bentonite clay to measure it. It's a technique they affectionately refer to as the bentonite method (Downing, Stranieri, and Strauss 1982).

Another science-y reason bentonite clay is especially good at healing breakouts is because it carries a strong negative charge, which is said to bond with the positive charge in many toxins. The toxins I've seen don't have their electrical charges listed on the ingredient label (*of course*), but I found NWCag's YouTube video to be compelling evidence that this line of reasoning is worth further investigation. In the video, he connects two wires to the positive and negative charges on a battery,

---

*Given the electrical charge of bentonite clay, it is advised that metal not be used when mixing the ingredients of your clay mask. I admit I don't fully understand why, but I use a glass dish and a plastic spoon just to be on the safe side.

and then places the other end of each wire into a beaker of bentonite clay mixed with water.* When he removes the wires from the clay, the negatively charged wire comes out clean, but because opposite charges attract, the positively charged wire is covered in a clump of clay. Is that not the wildest YouTube video you've ever heard of?

There could be some video-editing sleight of hand going on here, but NWCag doesn't seem like that kind of guy. He seems like the kind of guy who is affiliated with the agricultural program at Northwest College in Powell, Wyoming, and likes to post videos online about geology exercises (32 views), fertilizer calculations (152 views), and soil bulk density (2,180 views—*go Trappers!*).

Now feels like a good time to remind you that you don't need to use any of these treatments to maintain clear skin. If you heal your acne by avoiding fluoride, there won't be any breakouts to treat. Once I learned how to eliminate excess fluoride from my diet, clear skin became effortless.

My current skincare routine is a variation of the "caveman regimen" featured on The Love Vitamin, a website created by Tracy Raftl to help women heal their acne naturally.† It involves not washing or using any products on your face *at all*. I did not intentionally decide to do this method of skincare, rather I happened into it a few months ago when I temporarily moved to a fluoridated neighborhood. At first, I took the time to wash my face with spring water, but now that I'm writing this book, I spend every moment of my free time with you (totally worth it). Superfluous activities like face washing have fallen to the wayside, along with makeup applying, hair doing, jewelry wearing, shoe shopping, and a few other borderline nonessential activities I prefer not to mention. Like eyebrow tweezing. (Melissa, *just stop.*)

Every few days, I use a strigil-like tool in the shower to exfoliate my face. Since my skin is already soft from the shower, I don't even need to apply oil beforehand, although I do rub a few drops in afterward. Other

*To view the video, visit www.HiddenCauseofAcne.com/bentonite-clay
†See "Am I Still Doing the Caveman Regimen? (Three & a Half Years Later)" by Tracy Raftl at http://thelovevitamin.com/17857/am-i-still-doing-the-caveman-regimen

than that, my skin is completely free to do its own thing. I miss my saunas and clay masks because they feel good and make my skin glow, but this conversation with you is so much more important than that.

So there you have it. The skincare products I relied on to heal breakouts fast are: dirt, sweat, and oil. Oh, and a cup. How ironic is it that the primary villains in dermatologists' story of acne ended up being the solution they've been looking for all along? Who would have guessed, right? I mean, other than people who write Disney movies. And people who watch Disney movies. And all of antiquity. And the Big 4 Moms: Mother Nature, Mrs. McConaughey, Mrs. Potts, and Mommypotamus.*

---

*Visit www.HiddenCauseofAcne.com/guides to receive a one-page Quick Guide on how to heal breakouts overnight.

Under the Skin

Seaweed mask is always greener
On somebody else's face
You see doc to make skin clearer
But that is a risky place
Just look at the world around you
Right here in the human pore
Such wonderful things swim 'round you
What more is you lookin' for?

Under the skin
Under the skin
Darling it's better
Be a trendsetter
Oil that grin
There at the doc's they make you pay
To pop the pills (don't work anyway)
While lymph devotin'
Full time to floatin'
Under the skin

Down here all the lymph is happy
They swim, they are never bored
The lymph at the doc's ain't happy
They sad 'cause they is ignored
But lymph that's ignored is lucky
They in for a worser fate
One day when the pills get yucky
Guess who gon' feel des-o-late

Under the skin
Under the skin
Nobody bug us
Charge us and drug us
Gimme some fin
We what the doctor love to lance
Under the skin lymph love to dance
We got no troubles
Lymph flow like bubbles
Under the skin

Under the skin
Under the skin
When the whitehead
Begin to turn red
Lymph fixes my chin
What do they got? A lot of creams
We got the big ocean of our dreams
Each little zit here
Know when to quit here
Under the skin
Each little pimple
Lymph make it simple
Under the skin
All of that acne
It don't attack me
Lymph flow like lava
Only it's hotter
Ya we in luck here
Down in the muck here
Under the skin

6

Becoming Acne-Proof

You are braver than you believe, stronger than you seem, and smarter than you think.

CHRISTOPHER ROBIN

THERE IS ONE MORE SOURCE of fluoride you are exposed to that we did not discuss yet. It is the least understood but the most important. As you will soon see, it could possibly explain one of the fundamental mysteries of a little phenomenon we refer to as human civilization, amongst other stuff. I didn't include it in chapter 4 because it's not a source of fluoride you can avoid. You are exposed to it every day. All day. Even while you sleep. There is no getting away from it. Like the great poet Beyoncé says, nobody frees you from your body.

If you grew up consuming the typical industrialized diet—drinking fluoridated water, eating factory-farmed poultry, and snacking on raisins to your little heart's content—then by now your body itself is a significant source of fluoride. As we have learned, fluoride accumulates in human bone, teeth, and other tissues. It is unknown how long fluoride remains in the body, but a 2006 report from the National Research Council (NRC) references a half-life of twenty years for fluoride contained in human bone. That means it takes *twenty years* for just *half* of the fluoride you absorb into your bones today to be removed from your body.

The NRC admits this estimate might not reflect the true half-life of fluoride. There are so many variables involved that researchers are unable to determine the standard time frame it takes for fluoride to be eliminated from human tissue. Admittedly, they have not tried very hard. The CDC only recently began considering limited fluoride analysis in its national biomonitoring surveys.

But we don't need to know the average half-life of fluoride. I can think of many questions that are more helpful than trying to ascertain a national average. For example, what is the mechanism that causes the human body to eliminate fluoride? What other factors are involved? Is there a way to accelerate the process? Does fluoride cause the same symptoms on the way out as it does on the way in? If so, how can those symptoms be ameliorated?

There is a paucity of information on how to detoxify fluoride, but my obsessive intelligence analyst brain would not let me rest until I figured it out. Piecing together information gleaned from online forums, Internet, and small pockets of researchers in India, China, Africa, Canada, and here in the United States, a general framework for how to detoxify fluoride from living tissue starts to become apparent.

The most important data, of course, is how this information influences bodies in the physical world. I will tell you my experience with fluoride detoxification, but because this topic is so poorly studied, you will have to make some important decisions on how and if you will venture down this path.

It is possible to heal acne completely simply by avoiding certain foods and beverages. If that is your health goal, there is no need to proceed further. Case solved. But for me, after I realized my acne (and depression) was caused by fluoride, I started wondering if it was possible to eliminate enough fluoride from my body so I would no longer be sensitive to it. If I reduced the amount of fluoride in my body, would I be acne-proof? I also started wondering what other health effects I might experience in the future from fluoride that had already bioaccumulated in my bones, teeth, pineal gland, and who knows where else. Am I at a higher risk for arthritis? Cancer? What about my unborn children? Would it affect them? These questions were too important to let them linger. It was not easy, but I had to find answers. And find answers, I did.

THE MAGIC DRAGON
WHO LIVES BY THE SEA

My first lead came from a mysterious commenter who left a recommendation on my blog that I should investigate the work of a small group of physicians collaborating on an initiative they referred to as "The Iodine Project." I had just started writing about fluoride-induced acne and, as the commenter explained,

> Since we get so little iodine in our diets these days (unless you're into seaweed) we can start getting toxic build-ups of both fluoride and bromide in our systems—and both of these are toxic to our bodies. Dr. Guy Abraham has found that by increasing one's iodine intake, the body starts to flush out the bromide and fluoride, and the iodine takes up its proper place in its receptors. There are studies by Dr. Guy Abraham posted on the web, which include graphs of the results.

I found one of Dr. Abraham's graphs about fluoride. It is a simple chart that shows urinary fluoride levels for each of six patients before, during, and after thirty days of supplementation with 37.5 milligrams of iodine per day (Abraham 2005a). The fluoride levels were lowest prior to taking the supplement. On day one, they jumped to their highest point. On day thirty, they were lower than on day one, but still significantly higher than before the iodine supplement was taken. This general trend across all six subjects seemed to support Abraham's assertion that the iodine supplement was displacing fluoride. I was intrigued enough to investigate further.

Before vanishing into the digital ether, the mysterious commenter also mentioned that iodine is used to treat fibrocystic disease of the ovaries and breast, and that perhaps it affects cystic disorders of the skin in a similar fashion. Like the reproductive organs, skin requires a significant amount of iodine for optimal health.

In a lecture at the annual conference for the Association for the Advancement of Restorative Medicine in 2011, Jorge Flechas, a practicing family physician in North Carolina and one of the two doctors involved in the initial Iodine Project, explained that conventional medical opinion is fixated on the use of iodine by the thyroid gland and neglects its critical role elsewhere in the body.* He and the other "Iodine Doctors," as they have come to be known, noticed that when their patients' body tissues lack iodine, the result is cysts, nodules, scar tissue, and pain. It happens in the breasts. It happens in the muscles. And although Flechas doesn't mention acne, he does mention that 20 percent of the total iodine content of the body is contained in the skin.

Cysts, nodules, scar tissue, and pain. Does that sound familiar? When Flechas works with his patients to correct their iodine deficiencies through supplementation, these symptoms are resolved.

I see we have a few dermatologists in the crowd who are dying to employ an old doctor's tactic (you probably saw this one before) where they butt in on our conversation by tossing out some studies from the literature that supposedly disprove our burgeoning laymen theory that iodine is the ultimate antidote for acne. Even though dermatologists think diet does not cause acne, they almost unanimously agree that iodine *does* cause acne. They weasel around the diet connection because they only notice the phenomenon with iodine-based drugs and high amounts of seaweed that normal people don't eat, except for millions of people in other cultures who don't count for obvious reasons. (Just kidding, I don't know why. Is it racism?)

As early as the 1960s, dermatologists noticed this connection between iodine and acne (Hitch and Greenburg 1961). They still have not figured out how it works though, so we are going to have to explain

---

*View the lecture at www.HiddenCauseofAcne.com/Flechas

it to them. We should also give them a few tips for how they could have figured it out on their own by using some simple analytic techniques that professional analysts use to conduct analysis.

So, dermatologists are in widespread agreement that iodine can cause acne. That's great! Now let's see if we can find any disconfirming evidence to help them grow their assessment. As I mentioned in the introduction, the CIA textbook on *Psychology of Intelligence Analysis* by Richards Heuer is required reading for intelligence analysts during basic training. It should be required reading for medical researchers too. From chapter 4, "Strategies for Analytical Judgment": "An optimal analytical strategy requires that analysts search for information to disconfirm their favorite theories, not employ a satisficing strategy that permits acceptance of the first hypothesis that seems consistent with the evidence."

In intelligence analysis, analysts are instructed to intentionally look for disconfirming evidence and then not disregard it. Managers are advised to encourage dissenting viewpoints through devil's advocate exercises, interdisciplinary brainstorming, competitive analysis, intra-office peer review, and elicitation of outside expertise. They don't always do this (you know what they say—bureaucrats will be bureaucrats), but at least they are told that they should. I don't see that happening in government-sanctioned medicine where the stakes are magnified by the millions. This uncomfortable space of cognitive dissonance is where the analytic magic happens. It's what pushes us forward, forcing us to confront our misperceptions, refine our theories, and *learn* about the world.

Looking through the literature, it appears there are only a few researchers who put up any kind of fuss about iodine causing acne. In 1961, about ten years after most cities in North Carolina started fluoridating their water supply, two researchers from the University of North Carolina conducted a study to compare the rates of acne between adolescents who eat a lot of seafood on the coast, and those in the mountainous western region of the state where a diet rich in seafood, and therefore, iodine is less common (Hitch and Greenburg 1961). The results of their study were not what anyone expected. The adolescents who consumed more iodine had *less* acne.

The researchers concluded that iodine does not cause acne, but everyone else pretty much ignored them because iodine-induced acne was already confirmed, and who cares about dietary causes of acne anyway. If the researchers allowed for a period of cognitive dissonance rather than drawing the hasty conclusion that iodine doesn't cause acne, they might have focused follow-up studies on trying to figure out why iodine seems to cause acne in some people but inhibits acne in others.

This observation is easily explained within the fluoride theory of acne. As Guy Abraham's studies show, the ingestion of dietary iodine causes fluoride to be released in urine. If iodine turns out to be the antidote for acne, as I am proposing here, then consuming iodine on a regular basis would help limit the amount of fluoride that accumulates in your body, making you less susceptible to acne. However, if your body already contains significant amounts of fluoride and then you consume a large dose of iodine, the amount of fluoride released back into your circulation can cause acne just as it does when you consume too much fluoride in a glass of water.

My anecdotal experience with iodine supports this theory. I developed breakouts from seaweed, fish eggs, and iodine supplements. I never had a reaction from fish or shellfish, which contain significantly less iodine than seaweed.

Another piece of disconfirming evidence that iodine causes acne was uncovered in a 2007 article by William Danby from Dartmouth Medical School when he pointed out that iodine might not cause "true acne" because "the hallmark of acne, the comedo, is not part of the initial lesion." *Comedo* is the Latin term formerly used for flesh-eating worms, but dermatologists stole it to use as their secret code name for blocked pores since blackheads remind them of little black worms secreting from your skin.

The initial acne caused by iodine doesn't have a blocked pore. It's just pus (Jackson 1974). This observation disconfirms the widely held theory that acne is caused by clogged pores, but it makes perfect sense in our theory that acne is caused by fluoride. If dermatologists had pursued this piece of evidence, they might have been forced to admit that clogged pores are correlated with acne, but they do not cause it.

So how much iodine does it take to displace fluoride from your body? Oh boy, does that question open a can of comedones! The government's Recommended Dietary Allowance of iodine is 150 to 290 micrograms per day. The Iodine Doctors argue the optimal dose is roughly *one hundred times* that amount, and often higher if your body is storing toxic halides such as bromide and fluoride.

Of all the competing arguments in modern medicine, this is one of the most controversial ideas I've encountered. Mainstream physicians will tell you this amount of iodine can kill you, or at least permanently damage vulnerable thyroid tissue. Even some of my favorite "alternative" health docs such as Joseph Mercola and Chris Kresser are wary of recommending this amount of iodine in the absence of further studies. Paleo dieters conclude this amount of iodine wasn't a traditional part of the Paleolithic diet and is therefore undesirable.*

Real-world experiences of people supplementing with iodine don't help to clarify the matter. When Sally Fallon of the Weston Price Foundation and Katie from Wellness Mama tried iodine supplementation, they both experienced negative reactions and decided iodine was not right for them.

And yet, the Iodine Doctors point out that iodine supplements were widely consumed in these amounts since the discovery of iodine two hundred years ago. Moreover, they successfully treat thousands of patients in their clinics through iodine supplementation each year and are easily able to measure fluoride and bromide released in urine after iodine is ingested. Thriving communities of iodine discussion forums

---

*In intelligence analysis, we call this logic "mirror-imaging," where your assessment of how other cultures think and behave is unduly influenced by underlying assumptions of how people in your own culture think and behave. More on this later.

on Yahoo and Curezone support their claims as people share their experiences of how iodine healed various health crises.

How do we reconcile these viewpoints that seem to exist in direct conflict with each other? From chapter 8 of *Psychology of Intelligence Analysis:* "Analysis of competing hypotheses (ACH) requires an analyst to explicitly identify all the reasonable alternatives and have them compete against each other for the analyst's favor, rather than evaluating their plausibility one at a time." Brainstorming a variety of alternative hypotheses for a certain scenario is a handy way to become aware of possibilities you might not otherwise consider. Let's try it.

What are some of the possible hypotheses with regard to the safety of iodine supplementation? It is possible the official view of iodine is correct and amounts over 1 milligram are potentially dangerous. Another hypothesis is that the Iodine Doctors are correct, and the body requires 13+ milligrams for optimal health. A third option is that neither of them are correct. Maybe amounts over 1 milligram aren't dangerous, but the human body does not need that much iodine anyway. A fourth option is that they are both correct: amounts of iodine over 1 milligram are potentially dangerous, but the body requires 13+ milligrams for optimal health. Are you feeling some cognitive dissonance with that last one? That's a good sign.

Keeping these competing hypotheses in mind, we can now move on to the evidence. And not just the scientific evidence. Restricting our assessment to the scientific evidence would severely limit our analysis. From fluoridation to acne to raisins to mink oil, the controversies we covered in this book provide a game plan for how to approach this type of hazy health information. First we look at tradition and the historical precedent. How were people using iodine prior to the modern era when bureaucrats and billion-dollar industries gained a virtual monopoly on scientific consensus? Next, how did the tradition change? Who were the players involved and what were the stakes? By studying the story of iodine, we understand the science in context.

Iodine was discovered in 1811 when a Frenchman was creating potassium nitrate to make gunpowder during the Napoleonic wars.

The customary French method for making potassium nitrate was to use wood ash mixed with feces and urine and to let it decompose for a year. Excrement was abundant in Napoleonic France, but after several years of war, wood ash was scarce, so French manufacturers started burning seaweed instead.

One such Frenchman, a prior pharmacist and chemist named Bernard Courtois, was investigating corrosion on his copper vessels when he noticed that sulfuric acid added to seaweed ash gave off a plume of violet vapor that condensed as solid crystals the color and luster of graphite. When substances transition directly between gas and solid forms like this, without an intermediate liquid state, it is known as a process called sublimation.* The mysterious element was given the name iodine from the Greek word *ioeides,* meaning "violet colored."

Soon after he discovered iodine, Courtois began discussing the element with his pharmacist friends and provided samples for them to study. In less than a decade, physicians throughout Europe were using iodine to treat a common condition called goiter, an enlargement of the thyroid gland that was previously treated with burnt sea sponges. Iodine quickly earned a reputation for healing a variety of other ailments, from asthma and ulcers to joint disease and deafness. It proved to have seemingly miraculous antiseptic properties too. Gauze strips saturated in iodine were hung from the crossbeams in European hospitals. Seaweed was strewn across the floor. People wore small vials of iodine around their necks and Civil War soldiers carried iodine canteens as an essential part of their gear. In a letter to his brother, Vincent van Gogh raved about iodine as a treatment for syphilis.†

By the twentieth century, iodine was widely known as a panacea. Albert Szent-Gyorgyi, the Nobel Prize–winning physiologist who dis-

---

*Corroded copper vessels, a flash of a violet vapor, sublimation, lustrous crystals—how is chemistry *not* magic?

†For an interesting account of the history of iodine, see Lynne Farrow's book, *The Iodine Crisis: What You Don't Know About Iodine Can Wreck Your Life* (New York: Devon Press, 2013).

covered vitamin C in the 1930s, described iodine as "the universal medicine." In his biography, he even quotes a little rhyme that was commonly repeated about potassium iodide in medical school, "If you don't know what, where, or why, prescribe ye then K and I." Potassium iodide is the most popular form of iodine, especially a liquid solution called Lugol's that is still available today.*

By the 1920s, scientists were in agreement that not only does iodine heal goiter, but it also prevents it. It seems obvious now, but the idea that iodine deficiency leads to goiter was suggested throughout the previous century and repeatedly rejected because measuring methods for determining the iodine content of food, soil, and other relevant substances were new and untrusted, making it difficult to prove that iodine deficiency was the culprit. Many researchers at the time favored the idea of a "toxic agent" to explain the cause of goiter. What no one seemed to realize is that these two theories are not mutually exclusive.

In 1924, the United States began a salt iodization program in Michigan, the future birthplace of fluoridation and the heart of the American "goiter belt," which is comprised of the Great Lakes, Appalachia, and the Northwest. During World War I, Michigan doctors demonstrated that in some parts of the state, as many as 60 percent of men eligible for the draft had enlarged necks due to goiter, many of whom were disqualified from the military as a result (Leung, Braverman, and Pearce 2012). After iodine was added to salt, the incidence of goiter plummeted.

Iodine's popularity in the first half of the twentieth century is hard to imagine today. South Carolina license plates proudly displayed the phrase "The Iodine State" because of the high iodine content of the soil there. Championship swimmers preferred pools treated with iodine over those with chlorine (Abraham 2004). By mid-century, iodine was added to baked goods as a dough conditioner. A single slice of bread contained

---

*The term *iodide* refers to the ion form of iodine, meaning it is bonded with another element. To keep things easy, I will refer to the various types of iodine simply as iodine.

the full Recommended Dietary Allowance of 150 micrograms of iodine. Combined with iodine from eggs, milk, vegetables, seafood, and iodized salt, it becomes clear that many Americans were consuming much more than the recommended amount. Doctors treating patients with asthma described 300 *milli*grams of iodine as a "low" dose, and often used doses in the gram amounts on large numbers of patients for several years at a time with good results (Bernecker 1969; Abraham 2004).

Within a few decades, iodine was quietly removed from baked goods. We have since forgotten it can be used to treat swimming pools. Few people store a bottle of it in their bathroom cabinet these days, let alone around their neck. And when doctors don't know what, where, or why, no one ever told them to prescribe K and I.

This brings us to our next question. In the latter half of the twentieth century, why did a genuine essential nutrient that was so highly regarded since its discovery suddenly vanish from our doctors' medicine bags? What changed the historical precedent? To be honest, I'm tired of writing about bureaucrats and their institutionally entrenched viewpoints, and I am already *freaking out* over our grand finale later in this chapter. As much as I want to skip ahead, this part of the story is vital. We need to know where we came from to understand where we are. And we need to understand where we are before we can figure out how to get where we want to go.

Okay, where were we? I have a feeling we were about to discuss another old white guy. Oh right, Theodore Kocher. He was a physician and professor for forty-five years at the University of Bern, one of the five university hospitals in Switzerland. Kocher somehow dodged all the malpractice lawsuits he likely encountered while experimenting with thyroidectomies in the late nineteenth century and instead won the Nobel Prize in 1909 for his surgical techniques that reduced the mortality rate of thyroid surgery.*

---

*Just spitballing here, but perhaps he was able to maintain his reputation by taking credit for the discovery that the full thyroidectomies he pioneered result in cretinism. Kocher published an article on the topic in 1883 while failing to acknowledge the Swiss researchers

Kocher was the first surgeon to ever win the Nobel Prize and was considered a leading figure in the field of surgery at the time. He was also an outspoken critic of the use of iodine to treat patients with hyperthyroidism. Not surprisingly, he endorsed the technique he developed for thyroid surgery instead. Because of his influence in the medical community, many thyroidologists stopped using iodine for goiters associated with hyperthyroidism, and it ceased to even be a topic of discussion within the Royal Society of Medicine.

After Kocher's death in 1917, physicians at Mayo Clinic and elsewhere started reporting high success rates using Lugol's solution for hyperthyroid patients, and thus its reputation was reinstated (Abraham 2004). Iodine narrowly escaped vivisection from the Swiss master surgeon, but the field we would soon come to know as "modern medicine" had another hitman waiting in the laboratory wings.

Jan Wolff was a young undergraduate student when he joined Israel Chaikoff's laboratory at University of California at Berkeley in the mid-1940s. In 1948, with Chaikoff as a coauthor, Wolff published a short paper entitled, "The Inhibitory Action of Iodide upon Organic Binding of Iodine by the Normal Thyroid Gland." The whole article was less than two pages long, but its main assertion is still screwing with humanity's hormones today.

In the study, Wolff injected rats with varying dosages of potassium iodide labeled with a radioisotope of iodine discovered at Berkeley a few years prior. Over the next fifty hours, he observed how the iodine was absorbed by the rats' thyroid glands by removing them at designated intervals, grinding them up in a miniature rat thyroid blender, and then measuring their iodine content with a Geiger-Muller counter. In their seminal 1948 paper, Wolff and Chaikoff concluded, "thyroid tissue is inhibited by iodine regardless of its state of activity." Unlike Kocher, Wolff wasn't just referring to cases of overactive thyroid glands. He was

---

(cont.) who published a paper on the same condition the year prior and first reported it to him in 1872. (Type a search of "Emil Theodore Kocher" on Wikipedia. You'll see.)

referring to thyroid glands in general. The takeaway from his article was that "excess" iodine inhibits the thyroid's ability to produce thyroid hormone.

Another principle from Richards Heuer's *Psychology of Intelligence Analysis* is called for here. Like a well-crafted haiku, its words are simple but compelling. From chapter 6, "Keeping an Open Mind": "The principle of deferred judgment is undoubtedly the most important."

If a Berkeley grad student wants to inject perfectly congenial rodents with radioactive iodine and then put their thyroids in a blender to measure the iodine content, fine. (It's not actually fine, but we really don't have time to get into that here.)* But would it not be prudent to defer judgment on the dramatic conclusion that iodine, an essential nutrient, inhibits healthy thyroid function until more information can be gathered? Such as, what happens with continued iodine exposure after fifty hours? Do injections with radioactive iodine produce a different effect than forms of dietary iodine? Is decreased absorption of radioactive iodine a bad thing? And do these fluctuations in thyroid hormone make the rat *feel bad*?

No, Wolff and Chaikoff do not identify any of these intelligence gaps in their article. Instead they declare, and I repeat, "Thus thyroid tissue is inhibited by iodine regardless of its state of activity." The young Wolff draws that judgment right there in his very first paper on iodine supplementation. Such a dramatic statement turned out to be a great career move, but what would it mean for the rest of humanity?

Wolff continued to study the thyroid gland throughout his long and illustrious career in endocrinology, but as the bottom line of his 1948 paper revealed, he already made a hasty judgment. Once that mental model is in place, it is difficult to see the world any other way. As Heuer explains, "whether it manifests itself as self-censorship of one's

---

*See www.washingtonpost.com/national/health-science/a-new-model-of-empathy-the -rat/2011/12/08/gIQAAx0jfO_story.html

own ideas or fear of critical evaluation by colleagues or supervisors . . . [n]ew ideas are, by definition, unconventional, and therefore likely to be suppressed, either consciously or unconsciously."

Here is where Wolff and the endocrinology community in general make another big analytic error. Instead of looking for disconfirming evidence to grow their understanding of how iodine affects the thyroid gland, they focus on evidence that confirmed the hasty judgment that was already made. They noticed that in communities where salt iodization programs were established to prevent severe iodine deficiency, there was a rise in a certain form of hyperthyroidism (Stanbury et al. 1998). That evidence fits nicely into their theory, so they used it to justify their preexisting belief that iodine inhibits thyroid function.

They also noticed that the rate of hyperthyroidism sometimes dropped below previous levels after a few years of salt iodization, as was the case in Switzerland in the 1980s, and that increases in dietary iodine other than from iodized salt sometimes do not result in more reports of hyperthyroidism, as was the case in the United States in the 1960s (Stanbury et al. 1998). This evidence does not fit with their theory, so most endocrinologists mention it only in passing, if at all, missing out on a valuable opportunity to refine their current understanding of the world.

If endocrinologists had allowed disconfirming evidence about iodine into their analysis, they might have eventually realized that other variables influence how iodine affects the thyroid gland, such as the presence of nutritional cofactors and goitrogens like fluoride. Instead they cling to an oversimplistic theory developed by the big bureaucrat on campus while he was still in graduate school.

Wolff's theory that iodine inhibits healthy thyroid function came to be known as the Wolff-Chaikoff effect and is still seen as a major regulator of thyroid function. In 1969, Wolff published a review of all the evidence that confirms his theory on the pharmacologic effects of excess iodine. He proposed that the estimated daily iodine requirement "for man" (*eye roll*) is only 200 micrograms since that is the amount he suggests is required by the thyroid gland.*

The Wolff-Chaikoff effect is the reason iodine was removed from baked goods. It is the reason the American Thyroid Association issued a statement in 2013 warning against iodine consumption greater than 1 milligram, a small fraction of what many societies healthier than ours consume on a daily basis. It is also the reason the Recommended Dietary Allowance for iodine is 150 micrograms instead of the amount the human body needs to avoid iodine deficiencies other than simple goiter.

Since Wolff is an endocrinologist with a specialty in issues of the thyroid gland, he does not consider the iodine requirement of other organs. But how much iodine is needed by the ovaries, breasts, muscles, skin, and other essential body parts? The National Institute of Health's Endocrine Biochemistry Section, which Wolff directed as recently as 2008, has no idea because they never conducted those studies.

Wolff's half-century tenure as a government bureaucrat at NIH is an important part of our story. The National Institute of Health is the largest biomedical research agency in the world. It spends over $30 billion on medical research each year, most of which is awarded to universities, medical schools, and other research institutions around the globe. As you now know, Wolff—one of the founding members of the endocrinology branch at NIH who worked his way to chief of the Endocrine Biochemistry Section—established his very name and reputation on the Wolff-Chaikoff effect, which was used to denigrate iodine. If you were an endocrinologist seeking funding for your research, would you choose to investigate the validity of the Wolff-Chaikoff effect by studying the benefits of an inexpensive, nonpatentable nutritional supplement?

There's another reason the Wolff-Chaikoff effect is still standing.

---

*"Since the normal human thyroid gland delivers about 65 micrograms of organic iodine (T3 and T4) to the circulation per day, and since the iodide clearance of the thyroid is half that of the kidneys, a rough estimate of the daily iodide requirement for man would be about 200 micrograms of iodine per day. Approximately 10 percent of this is derived from deiodination of secreted organic iodine and the remainder from the diet" (Wolff 1969).

It's soooo cliché, you probably already know the gist of this story, but we should still get it all out in the open, so . . . Guess who was behind the denigration of dietary iodine. Dentists? Good guess, but no. It was another one of our story's big villains. The reason the Wolff-Chaikoff effect gained traction like it did was because of the drug lords, of course, and I'm not referring to dermatologists this time.

When Wolff started studying iodine in the mid-1940s, researchers were investigating a relatively new approach to treating hyperthyroidism. Instead of nourishing an unhealthy thyroid gland with seaweed or iodine as was the practice since the dawn of recorded history (and probably prior), doctors began attacking overactive thyroid glands with goiter-causing substances, known as goitrogens, in an effort to force them to stop overacting and behave as good little thyroids should.

Two such "antithyroid" medications, thiourea and thiouracil, were introduced in 1943 by a Harvard researcher named E. B. Astwood. These goitrogens would later evolve into the family of thionamides that doctors employ to assail thyroid glands today, such as methimazole (brand name Tapazole) and propylthiouracil. Wolff's paper was published five years after Astwood introduced these antithyroid medications to the world.

Wolff's study involved rats, as we know, but less than one year later, in 1949, Malcolm Stanley from Tufts University published a study extending the Wolff-Chaikoff effect to humans. This study was the evidence NIH pointed to in the 1960s when they figured out bakeries were using iodine as a dough conditioner and first expressed concern that it was significantly adding to the total dietary intake of iodine for most Americans (London, Vought, and Brown 1965). By the 1970s, bread manufacturers began using bromide in place of iodine.

As you might recall from our periodic chart, bromide is a halogen that sits above iodine on the table of the elements. Like fluoride, it is a known goitrogen that depresses thyroid function. Brominated flour has since been banned in Europe, Canada, Brazil, Argentina, Peru, China, South Korea, Sri Lanka, Nigeria, and probably a bunch of other

188 ⊗⊗ Affect (*v.*)

countries because *it causes thyroid cancer* (DeAngelo et al. 1998). In the United States, however, the FDA only "discourages" manufacturers from using brominated flour, which of course does not prevent it from showing up in your Tastykakes ("Five Controversial Food Additives" 2008).

It is unclear how Mr. Stanley was able to conduct human trials on the Wolff-Chaikoff effect, analyze the data, write a paper, submit it for publication, and have it published in a major medical journal only one year after Wolff's study was published. It is likely he had inside information about Wolff's line of research. There is nothing wrong with that, but it suggests there was some kind of relationship between the two researchers or that they worked together in some way. And who else did Stanley work with? E. B. Astwood, the man who introduced antithyroid pharmaceuticals just a few years prior.

Astwood and Stanley both worked at Tufts University at the time Stanley's paper extending the Wolff-Chaikoff effect to humans was published. Astwood is not listed as a coauthor on Stanley's paper, but in the requisite memoir written to enshrine his name in the community of science saints, Astwood's colleagues explain, "Because of his modesty, Astwood's name was withheld from many of the pioneering publications on the thyroid that came from his laboratory, even though he supplied the funds and space and contributed to the development of the ideas that generated the studies. Such self-effacement is uncommon among scientists" (Greep and Greer 1985). Astwood and Stanley authored another paper together that same year about using goitrogenic drugs as an alternative treatment to iodine for hyperthyroidism (Stanley and Astwood 1949).

Once the antithyroid drug manufacturers established their footing in the pharmaceutical world, there was no turning back from the Wolff-Chaikoff myth. As we've seen before, the industries that grow up around a government-institutionalized blunder serve as patrons for its propagation and sustainment. Like fluoridation and fluoristan toothpaste. Or vintage federal legislation and the beauty industry. Or the Raisin Reserve and puppy killers.

Thyroid medication is serious business. The hypothyroid drug levo-thyroxine, also known as Synthroid, is consistently listed as the most frequently prescribed pharmaceutical in the United States (Brown 2015). If a scientific consensus developed around the idea that thyroid disorders are best treated through increased consumption of iodine and decreased exposure to goitrogens, the industry would crumble. How could humble little iodine be expected to clear its name in the face of such a giant adversary?

Despite the government egos and industry interests vested in thyroid research, the occasional pro-iodine study still makes its way into the published literature. In 1993, Bill Ghent and his colleagues published a study in which 1,365 women with fibrocystic breast disease consumed 5 milligrams of dietary iodine per day for approximately one year. The results showed a significant reduction in fibrosis and no indication of the much-hyped Wolff-Chaikoff effect, even though Wolff predicted that daily amounts of iodine of only 2 milligrams were "excessive and potentially harmful" (Wolff 1969).

Like Wolff, Ghent was a bit of a bigwig himself—but in Canada where he served as Chairman of the Canadian Medical Association's Health Care Council. His article appeared in the *Canadian Journal of Surgery,* which helps explain why he was one of the few researchers to share the results of a study aboot "high dose" iodine supplementation, eh? Unfortunately for humanity, Ghent died three months before the study was published, leaving him little opportunity to promote his findings or conduct further investigation.

Guy Abraham, the professor of obstetrics mentioned earlier in this chapter, was retired and living the good life in California in the 1990s when he happened to read Ghent's paper on iodine supplementation a few years after it was published. He found it odd that Ghent reported such positive results with doses of iodine that were over twice as high as what American doctors were told was the safe limit. Abraham started researching the literature on iodine supplementation and found that studies were prolific prior to the 1940s, but mysteriously disappeared when goitrogenic drugs and a certain "famous thyroidologist" took the stage.

When Guy Abraham learned that 60 million people in Japan were eating iodine-rich seaweed every day without any indication of the Wolff-Chaikoff effect in action, he decided it was time to investigate the theory more directly. Using his own funding, he teamed with Jorge Flechas, the family physician in North Carolina mentioned earlier, to perform a few pilot studies and then a larger study of ten women to see if the results would confirm Ghent's observations (Abraham, Flechas, and Hakala 2002). They did, so he funded longer and larger studies, adding Michigan-based family physician David Brownstein to his team in the process. The Iodine Doctors did not see any signs of the Wolff-Chaikoff effect in their patients. Instead, all the evidence supported the hypothesis that the human body requires milligrams of iodine on a daily basis, not micrograms.*

I never met Guy Abraham to confirm this, but at this point of the story you can sense his blood pressure rising. He spent his whole career at UCLA studying women's health issues such as fibromyalgia and ovarian tumors. In the 1970s, he pioneered the development of methods to measure minute quantities of steroid hormones in biological fluids. In the 1980s, after realizing that premenstrual tension was an early indicator of more serious gynecologic disorders, he developed nutritional programs to alleviate PMS. So yes, Guy Abraham is a bona fide science saint. After realizing the entire population of women he was treating was iodine deficient for the sad reasons described in this chapter, and that simply correcting their iodine deficiency could lead to the resolution of many of the conditions he studied, Abraham felt **"grossly deceived"** by the national medical establishment he had been a part of for thirty-five years. (That's his bold print there, not mine.)

Guy Abraham was mad. And what happens when old, retired

---

*To see their full collection of published studies from 2002 to 2008, visit www.optimox .com/iodine-research

people get mad? Because I live in Florida, I know this one: they rant. It's *awesome.* Abraham published many articles in peer-reviewed journals throughout his career—*Obstetrics & Gynecology, The Journal of Reproductive Medicine, The Journal of Clinical Endocrinology & Metabolism, The American Journal of Clinical Nutrition,* and more. But in retirement, without an institution like UCLA attached to his name, he was able to spread his literary wings to really speak his mind.

Abraham started publishing research from his Iodine Project in a small natural health care journal called *The Original Internist.* As with the articles he wrote earlier in his career, they are still heavy on the science, but there's a distinct retiree tone that only people of a certain age can pull off. To give a few examples, Abraham documents a new condition called medical iodophobia where medicoiodophobes suffer from double standards, doublethink, doublespeak, and contradictory logic (Abraham 2006). He associates it with domestic bioterrorism and renames Wolff's theory "the Wolff-Chaikoff Iodophobic Domino Effect"* (Abraham 2005b).

Furthermore, each of his articles has as many as five exclamation points, sometimes two in a row. On occasion, he *might* use the word *zombifying* in place of "goitrogenic" and there are a few teeeeensy references to Lucifer, the flood, Adam and Eve, Old Testament Bible verses, and a link at the bottom of each article for a "Praise the Lord" 14" × 18" poster free of charge. So what? The man was clearly on to something.

But then in February 2013, Guy Abraham fell, hit his head, and made his quiet departure from the world. He didn't leave much information about himself behind. There are no "about me" pages or saccharine memorials written by his medical disciples. Judging from the lone black and white photograph posted of him online, that was probably the way he wanted it.

In generations past, Abraham's death might have spelled the end of his Iodine Project. But generations past didn't have a sidekick named

---

*I just noticed that abbreviates to Wolff-CIDE. Haha! Good one, Abraham.

Internet. She was smart enough to hold on to his articles. She also created a discursive space for people to share stories about his work. Then she sent a digital bird to whisper about it in my ear.

> *Today, the public relies heavily on the Internet for health information. . . . Control of health information on the Internet by iodophobic bioterrorists is a real threat to a population who depends on this source of information to make health-related decisions. Such a population is vulnerable and most likely will end up adopting iodophobic decisions to their detriment. . . . Iodophobic bioterrorism can be prevented through education of health care professionals and the public at large. Remember that the easiest and most effective way to destroy a nation is the removal of iodine from the food supply. Iodophobic bioterrorism is a real threat to our nation, and the enemies within our gates masquerade as guardians of our thyroid gland.*
>
> GUY E. ABRAHAM, 2005

HOW TO TRAIN YOUR DRAGON

The story of iodine described in the previous section is an edited version of its history. It can be no other way. But at least now you have an idea of how in the last two hundred years iodine was discovered, prized, vilified, forgotten, and then discovered again. We also learned it was widely used by doctors and individuals before government agencies endorsed pharmaceutical options in its place.

If you look closely at the history of iodine, you might notice that contemporary medical consensus is more a matter of the human story, not the science that scientists proclaim to have discovered. Who was promoted to a government soapbox? Whose studies support industry interests? Who died and stopped swaying scientific opinion in a certain direction or left behind a body of work unfinished? It will take a long time to develop a nuanced understanding of how these halogens affect the human body. If we want to be healthy now, we don't have time to wait for future generations to figure things out.

Now that we have a general understanding of the history of iodine research and the competing interests that brought our understanding of iodine to this point, we can move on to the most important question in our assessment of the conflicting health information surrounding iodine: what do our direct observations of the physical world tell us?

To answer this question for himself, Guy Abraham collaborated with two family physicians to incorporate iodine supplementation into their clinics. The Iodine Doctors put themselves at risk by including the use of iodine in their family practices while current medical opinion claims it is dangerous. They continue to do so because they see the dramatic positive effects iodine causes in their patients. Jan Wolff, on the other hand, spent his career experimenting in a laboratory. In his 1969 review detailing the effect of excess iodine, Wolff references 280 scientific papers, but he also notes, "The demonstration of the Wolff-Chaikoff effect in man remains presumptive." Scientists are not able to reproduce the negative effect of iodine in the laboratory without the use of goitrogens.

Like the Wright brothers and their airplane, the Iodine Doctors are at a great advantage in deciphering how the human body is affected by halogens because they are dealing with the human body directly in the physical world, not just in the abstract world of lab tests and scientific papers. We have that advantage too. These aren't studies that involve statistical analysis of rat thyroids and rabbit fur. Our tools and methods are much more direct than that. A glass of water, an iodine supplement, and a mirror will do. Patience and persistence are also helpful.

After learning how the Iodine Doctors use iodine to displace fluoride in their patients, I decided it was time to try it for myself. Like a kid trying to jump on a merry-go-round spinning just a little too fast, I fell on my face a few times when I first started increasing my iodine consumption. Because I don't want you to make the same mistakes I made, here are the biggest lessons I learned from my experience with iodine.

Lesson #1: Don't Start Here

Once you learn that iodine detoxifies fluoride, you might be tempted to rush out and buy some kombu or a bottle of kelp capsules and just see how things go. That is not a good idea. When I first started taking iodine, I was still in the phase where I was figuring out exactly how to avoid fluoride in my diet. My skin was mostly acne-free because I had cut out the major offenders, but there were still some sneaky sources of fluoride making their way in. This was not the appropriate time to throw a couple of kelp tablets into the mix, but that is what I did. It took longer than I care to admit to realize the kelp pills were causing more acne. I was so focused on rooting out fluoride, I nearly missed it. They also caused persistent water retention, especially around my upper abdomen. If you are going to attempt to detoxify fluoride, **wait until you completely heal your acne and you are confident you know how to limit your exposure to fluoride before adding iodine to your diet.**

Lesson #2: Food Isn't Always the Best Medicine

Since the kelp supplement didn't work out well for me, I returned to my old mantra of trying to obtain all the nutrients my body needs from food. I learned that fish eggs are nutrient-dense sources of iodine commonly eaten in traditional diets, so I started incorporating them into my breakfast each morning. Even the smallest of servings left me bloated and with breakouts. I tried seaweed snacks too, but had similar results. I eventually concluded that **food sources of iodine are not the best option for fluoride detoxification in fluoride-sensitive individuals** because it is nearly impossible to control the dose. As you will see, controlling the amount of iodine you consume is critical.

Lesson #3: Outsource

Next, I decided to try an actual iodine supplement. It was a very small dose, only slightly larger than the current Recommended Dietary Allowance. Again I developed acne and water retention, which this time spread to my calves. For the first time in my life, I woke up with an excruciating cramp in my left foot. I also developed heart palpitations. Reminder: I am demonstrating what *not* to do at home.

Effective iodine supplementation is more complicated than simply popping iodine pills. This is why all the books and articles you will read about iodine supplementation recommend that you **work with an "iodine-literate" health care practitioner** to safely use iodine to detoxify fluoride.* While that advice sounds reasonable, the problem is that there are not many "iodine-literate" health care practitioners out there. I could not find one within several hours' drive even though I was living in a major metropolitan center at the time, so I gave up on iodine and started pursuing another lead on fluoride detoxification.

Lesson #4: Beware of Imposters

Boron has also been found to detoxify fluoride, but I cannot recommend it. The research is sparse, but in one study from 1987, Chinese researchers used borax to treat thirty-one patients suffering from skeletal fluorosis (Zhou, Wei, and Ldu). After administering increasing doses of borax, they measured the fluoride in the patients' urine against that of a control group and concluded that borax is an effective way to eliminate fluoride. Other studies on rats (Marcovitch and Stanley 1942) and rabbits (Elsair et al. 1980; Elsair et al. 1981) draw the same conclusion. The online forum EarthClinic has a popular thread on using borax to detoxify fluoride, but I was skeptical of ingesting a substance I currently use to clean my toilet. Instead of borax, I tried a boron supplement. Even half the recommended dose resulted in acne and bloating, but then

---

*Lynne Farrow, founder of Breast Cancer Choices, a nonprofit organization dedicated to educating women about the use of iodine therapy, maintains a list of iodine-literate physicians on her website at www.breastcancerchoices.org/ipractitioners.html

I also developed abdominal cramping, nausea, diarrhea, weakness, and dizziness—all signs of acute fluoride toxicity.

I was smart enough to stop taking boron, but dumb enough to try it again on two separate occasions to verify it was the boron that caused my symptoms and not a virus or bacteria. Prunes contain unusually high amounts of boron, and I have found they can cause breakouts, bloating, and queasiness, especially motion sickness, if I eat too many. Raisins, dates, avocados, almonds, peanuts, and other nuts can also contain significant amounts of boron. I eat several of these foods on a regular basis and do not notice breakouts (perhaps it is a function of the cofactors?), but if you eat them in abundance, keep an eye out for signs of fluoride detoxification. Don't worry about memorizing this. It's all in the cheat sheet.*

Lesson #5: No Nutrient Is an Island

Returning to the iodine angle, I finally got serious about learning the details of iodine supplementation and read *Iodine: Why You Need It, Why You Can't Live Without It* by David Brownstein, one of the Iodine Doctors. I also read *The Iodine Crisis* by Lynne Farrow, founder of Breast Cancer Choices. Both authors emphasize iodine supplementation as part of a complete nutritional program.

When fluoride is released back into circulation, your body needs extra nutrients to help eliminate it safely. I assumed that relying on nutrient-dense foods would be enough, but a healthy diet did not sufficiently counterbalance the effects of fluoride detoxification. A. K. Susheela, a fluoride researcher in India, uses essential nutrients and antioxidants to reverse the effects of skeletal fluorosis (Susheela and Bhavnagar 2002). A traditional nutrient-dense diet is the best way to maintain good health, but to overcome fluoride poisoning, **an effective iodine supplementation program requires additional supplements including selenium, magnesium, vitamin C, and unrefined sea salt.**

---

*To receive a copy of the cheat sheet, see www.HiddenCauseofAcne.com/guides

Selenium is particularly important. In the iodine supplementation plan developed by the Iodine Doctors, these supplements are referred to as companion nutrients.

Lesson #6: What You See Is Not All There Is

I first took the iodine-loading test in 2010 when Hakala Research Laboratory agreed to provide a free test kit in return for an article about it on my blog. At the time, I had healed my acne by avoiding fluoride, but it was before I figured out how to increase my consumption of iodine. The test involves taking a 50-milligram iodine pill and then measuring the amount of iodine secreted in the urine for the next twenty-four hours. Working with their patients, the Iodine Doctors determined that iodine sufficiency is reached when the body eliminates 90 percent or more of the iodine pill within a twenty-four-hour period. The test can also measure how much fluoride and bromide is excreted in this same time frame.

According to my initial test results, my body eliminated 93 percent of the iodine pill. Hakala noted that a false high reading in your first test is a common result in people who have a "symporter defect" that causes iodine to not be properly absorbed by the cells. It typically resolves after several weeks of iodine supplementation. At 0.36 milligram, my fluoride level was among the lowest they had ever seen, which made sense since I had been avoiding fluoride for a couple of years. But if my body was not eliminating fluoride, why was I having such a negative reaction from iodine? After I took the 50-milligram pill, my skin broke out in a deep cystic welt but not until two days later. This fluoride would not have been captured in the twenty-four-hour screening.

I have taken the iodine-loading test multiple times in the last few years. As the lab predicted, my iodine results went down to 73 percent after I began taking a daily iodine supplement. But the fluoride measurements did not give an indication that a significant amount of fluoride was being released from my tissue. My bromide levels eventually decreased from 16 milligrams to less than 3 milligrams as measured in the twenty-four-hour urine screening, but the fluoride measurements stayed consistent at about 1 milligram. I even ordered fluoride tests for the day before and several days after taking the 50-milligram pill. My fluoride levels dipped slightly on the day the pill was taken but remained at 1.04 to 1.24 all the other days.

There are many potential explanations for why a sharp increase in fluoride is not measured in my twenty-four-hour iodine-loading test, but we are far from exploring them. We have barely begun to study these halogens, much less develop a deep understanding of all the intricate ways they interact with the human body.* The current medical research on halogens is oversimplified and unsophisticated. Most doctors still think fluoride's main effect is to prevent cavities. Studies don't differentiate between varying types of iodine. Seaweed is equated with iodine even though it contains many other chemical constituents, and the interaction of various goitrogens and important nutritional cofactors are almost completely neglected.

The Iodine Doctors seem to focus on bromide detoxification because that is what is reflected most in the twenty-four-hour iodine-loading test, but I suspect **our current understanding of iodine supplementation is missing an important part of the fluoride picture.** Bromide has been widely found in fire retardants, pesticides, fumigants, and electronics as well as brominated flour used in baked goods and brominated vegetable oils used in Mountain Dew and other toxic beverages. Most Americans have been exposed to significant amounts of bromide, but it's not as if they add it to the water supply and guilt you into brushing your teeth with it twice a day.

---

*My main theory at the moment is that perhaps this situation is similar to the case when researchers at the Medical College of Georgia were unable to detect the level of fluoride they suspected was contained in instant tea that was causing skeletal fluorosis in several patients. When they developed a new diffusion method for testing the fluoride content of tea, they found much higher fluoride levels than when they used the traditional electrode method. The Iodine Doctors use the electrode method for measuring the fluoride content of urine. But who knows, there are many other possible explanations.

Lesson #7: Bigger Isn't Always Better

When a job transfer took me to a new state, I finally lived within driving distance of one of the recommended "iodine-literate" doctors. I told him about my sensitivity to iodine, and after ordering the necessary tests to check my thyroid gland (it is important not to skip this step), he helped me get started on the iodine program. I began with just the companion nutrients, building up to the recommended dosages over a period of a few weeks. I was also sensitive to selenium, so I began with a quarter of the recommended dose and added another quarter each week, reaching the full dose after one month.

After everything checked out with my blood tests, the doctor suggested I start iodine supplementation with one drop of Dulse Liquid, which equates to 11 micrograms of iodine. I added one drop per day until I reached the full dose of 225 micrograms over a period of twenty days. I stayed there for two weeks before switching to a pill that contains 225 micrograms of potassium iodide. In the past, this amount of iodine caused my skin to break out, but **because I started with a minuscule dose and added to it in small increments over a long period of time, I was able to increase my iodine intake with minimal side effects.** I took the potassium iodide pill for one week and then added another pill each week until I was taking four pills, or 900 micrograms, of iodine per day.

The doctor recommended I continue taking four iodine pills per day until I finish the bottle and then switch to Iodoral, the pill form of liquid Lugol's solution, which was the iodine supplement of choice in the early twentieth century. Like Lugol's, Iodoral is a blend of potassium iodide and iodine. It is the supplement the Iodine Doctors use in their clinics since Lugol's can irritate the stomach and the taste is unpleasant to most people. The Iodoral tablet my doctor gave me was 12.5 milligrams, but he suggested I start with a half dose to see how my body reacted to it. My body reacted to it the same way it reacted to other large doses of iodine: acne, bloating, digestive problems, and heart palpitations. I tried cutting the pill in quarters and only taking it every other day, but it still did not go over well. My doctor proposed that some people just can't take larger doses of iodine and suggested I stick to 900 micrograms, which is still a significant increase from what most people consume.

The idea that my body was not able to handle milligram doses of iodine did not resonate with me. I saw another possible explanation. Perhaps the reason my body reacted negatively to Iodoral wasn't because it was simply too much iodine for my body to handle. Maybe it was because I tried to increase the dosage too quickly. Rather than jumping from 900 micrograms to 6 milligrams as my doctor originally recommended, I increased to 1, then 1.2 a few days later. Then 1.4 and so on.* It took a solid year, but eventually I was able to build up to the 50 milligrams prescribed in Dr. Brownstein's book on iodine. And since I increased the dose gradually instead of trying to jump ahead, I was able to do so without experiencing negative side effects. This was the most important lesson I learned from my experience with iodine supplementation. If you don't remember any of the other lessons, please at least heed this one: ***start low and go slow.***

I've been supplementing with 50 milligrams of iodine for almost eight months now. My iodine-loading test increased from 73 to 84 percent iodine saturation, and I am close to the 90 percent the Iodine Doctors note is correlated with optimal health.† More importantly, the positive changes in my mind and body corroborate that I am on the right track. Before taking iodine, I came home from work exhausted. I thought being tired after work was normal, but now I have energy to do yoga, take a walk with my husband, go to dinner with a friend, play with my dog, and generally live life outside of my 9 to 5 commitment.

The mental changes have been even greater. As someone who

---

*Visit www.HiddenCauseofAcne.com/guides to receive a one-page Quick Guide on my experience detoxifying fluoride with iodine.

†Update from the future: As I work on the final edits for this book prior to publication, here is a noteworthy development. After continuing on 50 milligrams of Iodoral for several more months, I retook the iodine-loading test. My iodine saturation was 100 percent and my fluoride levels tripled to over 3 milligrams.

thinks for a living, I can attest that iodine caused a sharp increase in my mental acuity. I did not notice the fog until it lifted. I am not under the delusion that my way of detoxifying from fluoride is the final way or the best way. It is possible that boron or cilantro or tamarind or fairy dust is more effective and causes fewer side effects. And certainly, there are secrets to iodine still to be uncovered.

We are only at the beginning stages of understanding halogens, but there is another reason I believe iodine is the key to unlocking the whole mystery. *Hal* is a word-forming element from Greek meaning salt or sea. *Gen* signifies giving birth to. In its most basic sense, the term halogen conveys the idea of giving birth to the sea. What a provocative notion considering the sea is what gave birth to all life as we know it.

As you can probably tell, there's a story here. It is reaching from beyond the ocean's edge to be told, pulling at me to assume the rule of storyteller with a timeless persistence I can't refuse. So grab a fluoride-free drink and a nutrient-dense snack, dim the lights, and settle in for what is sure to be a memorable tale as I present to you: the untold story of *Homo sapiens*.

THE LAND BEFORE TIME

We shall not cease from exploration, and the end of all our exploring will be to arrive where we started and know the place for the first time.

T. S. ELIOT

Analysis of intelligence failures reveal they are more commonly caused by flawed assumptions rather than flawed information. Relying on assumptions in analysis is unavoidable. Instead of trying to avoid assumptions, intelligence analysts are encouraged to try to make their assumptions as explicit as possible, stating them up front so they can be challenged and, if appropriate, disconfirmed. Assumptions that have the greatest impact on an assessment are called lynchpin assumptions. Challenging lynchpin assumptions is a valuable technique in moving an assessment forward.

It is not surprising that the government-sanctioned mainstream medical community is confused about the daily requirement for iodine, so I won't bother challenging their assumption that government-approved drugs are the answer to everything. But the alternative health community, for lack of a better term, is generally in agreement that nutrition is the key to health and that fluoride is a neurotoxin that depresses thyroid function. Yet many alternative health advocates are wary to endorse the milligram amounts of iodine that the Iodine Doctors claim are correlated with optimal health in their patients.

In a 2009 discussion about iodine, one of my favorite paleo bloggers, Stephan Guyenet, illustrates a lynchpin assumption of why milligram doses of iodine are not widely endorsed by the alternative health community. In the comments section of a blog post about iodine, a reader asks Stephan what he thinks about Dr. Abraham's iodine protocol. He replies that eggs and dairy can be a good source of iodine if the soil is not deficient, but he expresses suspicion of "anything outside of a natural range of intake."

One of the assumptions Stephan is making in his response is that the traditional *Homo sapiens* diet is an important guide for how we should eat today. Even though we are likely exposed to more toxic sources of fluoride and other goitrogens, I largely support that assumption, so I'm not going to challenge it here. Another assumption he makes is that milligram amounts of iodine are not native to the *Homo sapiens* diet. That's the one I am going to challenge. We are about to cover a lot of ground, so hold on tight. Here we go.

There are a number of techniques that can be used to challenge assumptions. The one I am choosing to use here is called "thinking backwards," also referred to as the "crystal ball" technique. Thinking backwards is an intellectual exercise that begins with an assumption contrary to the assumption you are challenging. For example, say you make an assumption that penguins are not capable of producing a nuclear weapon. In the thinking backwards exercise, you start with the assumption that penguins *are* capable of producing a nuclear weapon and then you think backwards to figure out what events had to occur a year ago (or a million years ago) to make that happen. It's as if you looked into a crystal ball and saw that in the near future penguins do in fact detonate an atomic bomb. Now your job as an analyst is to go back and put the pieces together that you missed the first time around.

By imagining an unexpected future event, you are forcing yourself to see the current situation differently. As Heuer explains in *Psychology of Intelligence Analysis,* "Analysts will often find, to their surprise, that they can construct a quite plausible scenario for an event they had previously thought unlikely. . . . This suggests your assumption is open to some question."

In our scenario, we look into the crystal ball and see that enlightened paleo dieters of the future conclude beyond question that daily milligram doses of iodine are—and always have been—a natural part of a healthy *Homo sapiens* diet. How did we miss that? We need to go back and put the pieces together. Starting with the present day, we now challenge ourselves to think back over time to figure out how humans could have become dependent on milligram doses of iodine.

If we are looking for evidence of significant consumption of iodine in a healthy human diet, we are not likely to find it in present-day populations. The current global prevalence of inadequate iodine consumption is widely recognized. The World Health Organization claims two billion people consume less than 100 micrograms of iodine per day, making iodine deficiency the single greatest cause of intellectual disability (de Benoist et al. 2008). Researchers in the *Lancet* estimate that 187 million people suffer from goiter due to a lack of dietary iodine, approximately 2.7 percent of the global population (Cos et al. 2012). Even cretinism, now referred to as congenital hypothyroidism, has been found to be on the rise in the last two decades in the United States, although it is now reversible when detected in early screenings (Olney, Grosse, and Vogt 2010).

To expand our search, a more fruitful approach is to study societies that still consume a traditional diet, where industrialized food corporations have yet to make their mark. Such societies are difficult to find today, but less than one hundred years ago that was not the case. Furthermore, we don't want to throw a dart at the map and study any nonindustrialized society—we want to find the healthiest ones and focus on those.

This next sentence might come as a shock. The best research I've found detailing the traditional diets of the healthiest human societies in the world came from a dentist. (*I know, right?*) His name was Weston Price, and he traveled the world in the 1930s looking for societies where tooth decay was rare. He found groups of people in Europe, Africa, Asia, Australia, and the Americas who displayed a remarkably high resistance to dental decay. But what was even more astonishing was that these same societies also seemed to be resistant to many of the health disorders plaguing the industrialized world, from tuberculosis and heart failure to cancer and varicose veins. Price concluded that dental decay is a symptom of deeper health problems caused by poor nutrition.

In his book published in 1939, *Nutrition and Physical Degeneration,* Price describes his travels to these societies and includes details of their traditional diets. He also includes photographs to demonstrate the dietary traditions that produce strong teeth, as well as the deleterious effects that result when native people switch to a diet of sugar, flour, and other modern foods. His book is compelling evidence that traditional diets are an effective way to prevent the so-called "diseases of civilization." But what can it tell us about iodine? If our crystal ball is correct, and for this exercise we must assume it is, then these healthy societies must have been consuming high amounts of iodine. Now it's our job to figure out how they could have done it.

Most of the groups Price describes in his book consume copious amounts of iodine-rich seafood. Traditional Polynesians, Melanesians, Aborigines, Eskimos, Gaelics, Native American Indians, New Zealand Māori, and Torres Straight Islanders all lived predominantly off the sea. Eskimos fed their children fish eggs as their first food after weaning and developed complex processes to turn kelp into dried cakes that could be stored and eaten during winter (Kuhnlein and Turner 1991). Pacific Islanders put an emphasis on shellfish and made great efforts to collect them in abundance, also eating a variety of seaweed as part of their regular diet. On the west coast of Scotland, a seaweed called dulse was eaten in a thick broth with oats or simply boiled and served with butter. Other types of seaweed were turned into sauces, soups, and puddings.

So many of the healthy societies Price encountered relied on seafood that he deliberately embarked on arduous travel inland with the hope of finding people without cavities who did not include food from the sea in their diet. He did not always succeed. When he visited Viti Levu, for example, the largest island in Fiji, he drove deep into the interior and then proceeded on foot but was disappointed by the piles of seashells that lined the path. His guide informed him that even during times of bitter warfare, the inland people found a way to trade with coastal rivals for essential foods from the sea. Several of Price's guides in the Pacific Islands revealed that a lack of essential seafoods for people living in the interior was the primary motivation for cannibalism. It was common knowledge that fishermen were "especially sought for staying a famine" because of the nutrients from the sea their bodies contained (Price 1935).

During his years of travel, Price did manage to find a few healthy societies who do not eat seafood. These are the groups that paleo dieters and traditional food enthusiasts use to demonstrate that the amount of iodine recommended by the Iodine Doctors is not a normal part of the *Homo sapiens* diet. But since our crystal ball already told us that these doses of iodine *are* required for optimal health, our challenge in this exercise is to figure out how these people could have obtained iodine without consuming food from the sea.

Next to seafood, the other major food group Price identifies as preventing dental decay is dairy. Is it a coincidence that next to seafood, the other major food source of iodine is dairy? Unlike fluoride, iodine is eagerly passed on to babies through mother's milk.

The best example from Price's book comes from the residents of a town in the Swiss Alps where the diet consisted largely of dairy products, rye bread, meat once a week, and some vegetables in the summer. Milk doesn't contain nearly as much iodine as seaweed, but the people Price encountered in the Swiss valley weren't your average milk drinkers. They were a little obsessed with it. Not only were dairy products their primary source of calories—a bowl of heavy cream was considered the quintessential health beverage—but they literally celebrated the presence of divinity in the June butter produced from cows grazing near the snow line in summer. (The ceremony involved lighting a wick in a bowl of butter and letting it burn in a special sanctuary, as one does.)

Early in Price's book, he comments that people previously believed a lack of iodine was the cause of the rampant dental decay in Switzerland, but he quickly dismisses this possibility. As Price explains, "That this is not the case seems clearly demonstrated by the fact that dental caries is apparently as extensive today as before, if not more so, while the iodine problem has been met through a reinforcement of the diet of growing children and others in stress periods with iodine in suitable form." *But Wes, what if iodized salt is only sufficient for preventing goiter and cretinism but not dental decay and other signs of physical degeneration?* He doesn't seem to consider that possibility. Later in the book, Price writes about the inadequacy of reinforcing the diet with a few synthetic products known to represent certain nutrients, but he never applies this point of view to iodized salt.

The Masai people in Africa are another group of dairy enthusiasts Price identifies as prime examples of robust health. They are even more serious about their cows than the Swiss group. When it comes to livestock, the Masai would be considered a little on the OCD side by our current standards. As Price explains, they carefully cultivate their herd by judging their cows on how quickly a calf starts running after it is born, which for a Masai calf is only a matter of minutes. The Masai's primary diet consists of milk, meat, and a few vegetables. When available, growing children and pregnant or lactating mothers receive a daily ration of raw blood. The iodine content of Masai cow blood is difficult to track down, but where there is thyroid hormone, there is iodine. Could blood have been the extra source of iodine that gave the Masai people their physical prowess?

The farther Price moved from the sea, the more resourceful and creative the people he studied seem to become with their diets. The First Nations of northern British Columbia and Yukon Territory were some of the most remote societies he visited. They did not have access to seafood, not even migrating salmon, and it was too cold for dairy or agriculture. Instead, they lived predominantly off wild game such as moose and caribou. This is the group Sally Fallon Morrell, President of the Weston Price Foundation, points to in her article, "The Great Iodine Debate," when she asserts that the amount of iodine consumed by the people Price studied is mostly in line with the current Recommended Dietary Allowance.* But our crystal ball already told us that the people in these healthy societies must be getting a hefty dose of iodine from somewhere. Does Price provide any clues as to where?

In his book, Price notes that the Inuit of the Far North live mostly off the organ meats of wild game, not the muscle meat as we prefer today. He even remarks on their ability to select certain organ meats and tissues to prevent specific diseases. At one point, he asks an older man in the group why his people do not suffer from scurvy, a disease caused by a lack of vitamin C. At first, the man says it is simply a white

---

*The reference Fallon Morell cites for the ranges of iodine reported in the diets of Inuit and Eskimos during Price's travels is a personal communication with Anore Jones, author of *Fish That We Eat*. (Jones's book, a 290-page tome on the diet of the Inupiat people in Northern Alaska, contains 374 references to fish eggs.) On her list of groups who consume seaweed as reported by Price, Fallon Morrell fails to include all the sea-bordering societies of the Pacific and instead highlights only the Gaelic peoples of the Outer Hebrides and the Andean Indians of Peru. See Sally Fallon Morrell, "The Great Iodine Debate," The Weston A. Price Foundation, June 22, 2009, www.westonaprice.org/modern -diseases/the-great-iodine-debate

man's disease (the ol' genetic argument—heard that one before), but after asking for permission from the chief, he tells Price their secret. When a family consumes a moose, they divide the two small balls above the kidneys so that each family member is given a share. These are the moose's adrenal glands, and as Price points out, they are the richest source of vitamin C in all animal or plant tissues.

What secret would the man have revealed if Price had asked about goiter? Do caribou, like cows, have an iodine recycling system in their oral-salivary and gastrointestinal tracts to protect them against low dietary iodine? If the Inuit ate these organs, how much iodine would they consume? The Inuit scrape every last morsel of bone marrow and emphasize its value for growing children. Does iodine, like fluoride, accumulate in bone? Or, perhaps the Inuit traded with coastal groups for dried kelp, as northern groups in British Columbia were known to do (Kuhnlein and Turner 1991).

Price does make a point to note how the native people of the Far North near the Arctic Circle worked to ensure adequate iodine intake for the segment of their population most vulnerable to iodine deficiency: newborn infants. Parents planning to conceive would eat the enlarged thyroid glands of male moose who came down from the high mountains during mating season. This explains why more children were born in the month of June than any other month.

Other inland groups were equally resourceful. In Africa, they made ant pies, mayfly pudding, and a type of flour from dried locusts. Price notes, "the natives of Africa know that certain insects are very rich in special food values at certain seasons, also that their eggs are valuable foods." Perhaps the people Price studied in Africa selected their insects based on their iodine content, like the inland people of Taxco, Mexico, do with stinkbugs (Sala 2013). Insect eggs were especially valued. Is it a coincidence that next to seafood and milk, eggs are known as a significant source of iodine? Inland Aborigines and Amazon Indians also included eggs in their diet whenever possible, particularly eggs from waterfowl and other birds. In the high Andes of Peru, Price found that people traveled hundreds of miles to gather fish eggs and dried kelp so they would not get "big neck" like the white people do. In Africa, goiter was treated with the ashes of iodine-rich water hyacinth and other plants that grew along the Nile River.

Because of the Humboldt Current and the extraordinary array of marine life it brings to the coast of Peru, Price was particularly interested in the ancient people who lived along the western coast of South America. In a study of 1,276 skeletal remains, he did not find a single deformity of the dental arches. Price laments that little is known about the ancient cultures that lived there, but he does tell us their modern counterparts emphasize the importance of fish eggs for the development of children, especially girls. The glands of a certain fish, the angelote, were consumed by young couples prior to conceiving. Weighing up to a pound each when dried, the male glands were a special food eaten by fathers-to-be to ensure healthy offspring.

Despite the large amount of fish eggs and seaweed Price encounters in his travels, he overlooks the importance of iodine, which he sees as a trace mineral the human body only requires in minute quantities. Instead, he attributes robust health primarily to large amounts of fat-soluble vitamins.* Price allows for much more sophistication in his conception of vitamins than with minerals, but iodine isn't exactly a vitamin or a mineral. As we discussed in chapter 3, it is a halogen.

Furthermore, it would take enormous effort to calculate the iodine content of the traditional diets Price studied to quantify their true values. Not only is it difficult to determine the iodine content of mayflies during a designated period in their mating season, but as we have seen time after time, the nutritional content of a specific food depends on a myriad of factors, making an established average little more than a vague suggestion.

For the average American, it might not be considered normal to

---

*I'm not saying his assessment is inaccurate, but I am saying that if our crystal ball turns out to be telling us the truth, then his analysis wrongfully neglects iodine and needs to be reworked in light of new information.

consume milligrams of iodine, but clearly "normal" is a matter of perspective. In most of the groups Price studied, the seaweed and fish eggs in their diet could easily provide daily doses of iodine in the milligram amounts. For the inland groups, it is possible their meticulous diets were intentionally constructed to be rich in iodine from dairy products, select organ meats, eggs, and other unconventional sources.

Continuing our exercise in thinking backwards, what about the first people in the Americas? Weren't they savage nomads running around spearing mammoths and mastodons for dinner? Price admits to knowing very little about the culture of the ancient people of South America. So did modern anthropologists until 1975, when a local farmer in a region of southern Chile called Monte Verde found a strange "cow bone" and showed it to a visiting veterinary student. The bone turned out to be from a mastodon, and it dramatically altered the prevailing view of the early peoples of the Americas.

It is difficult for archeologists to reconstruct a full picture of evolutionary diets from the bits of stone, bone, and teeth that remain in ancient ruins, but the Monte Verde site was special. When archaeologists excavated the region where the mastodon bone was found, they uncovered the remains of an ancient community that lived along the banks of Chinchihuapi Creek located 36 miles from the current Pacific coastline. Shortly after the region was originally occupied, the waters of the creek rose to form a peat-filled bog that inhibited the bacterial decay of organic material left at the site, preserving perishable artifacts for millennia.

What did archaeologists find amongst the wooden tools, scraps of leather, human footprints, and chunks of mastodon meat? Nine species of seaweed, along with a type of algae that grows exclusively on littoral rocks and trees. The seaweed was collected across a variety of regions and seasons. Because of its widespread dispersion in hearths and cooking areas throughout the site, archaeologists concluded it was used for both food and medicinal purposes. All nine species were found to be an excellent source of iodine (Dillehay et al. 2008).

There is another aspect of the Monte Verde site that made it special. Not only is it one of the rare open-air prehistoric communities found in the Americas, but when archaeologists dated the site they determined it is 14,800 years old—over a millennia older than the oldest known settlement in the Americas at the time. Many experts refused to accept the age of the Monte Verde site because they had already created a nice story depicting the first *Homo sapiens* crossing into the Americas after the retreating ice age opened the Bering land bridge from Siberia to Alaska 13,000 years ago. How could a band of *Homo sapiens* have settled in the southern tip of Chile 1,800 years *before* the land bridge opened?

Forced to reconsider their theory, some archaeologists proposed it was a coastal migration that brought *Homo sapiens* from Asia to the Americas. Instead of trekking to the New World across a land bridge on foot, they believe people sailed along the coast and quickly migrated all the way to the southern tip of South America by boat.

The coastal migration theory was a major departure from the previous view, but it steadily gained support as evidence mounted. Another important clue was unearthed in the mid-1990s when paleontologists were excavating an ancient bear den on the tip of Prince of Wales Island in southeastern Alaska. Contrary to previous views that these island chains were covered in glacial ice during the last ice age and uninhabitable, researchers uncovered animal remains indicating the cave was continuously inhabited for the past 40,000 years. Then in 1996, they found the bones of a 10,000-year-old *Homo sapiens,* the oldest human remains ever found in Alaska or Canada.

Even though the man's bones were found 300 miles inland where land meats were abundant, isotopic analysis revealed they have the signature of a seal or ocean fish, meaning the man's diet was almost exclusively from the sea. Stone tools made of a volcanic glass called obsidian were also found at the site. Archeologists conclude it was likely brought in by boat from Mount Edziza in British Columbia 150 miles away. The man's mitochondrial DNA matched forty-seven samples from American

Indians located down the western coast of the Americas, further supporting the idea of a rapid coastal expansion.

What started as a fringe theory in the 1970s went mainstream by 2007 when Jon Erlandson from the University of Oregon published his article, "The Kelp Highway Hypothesis" (Erlandson et al. 2001). Erlandson proposed that seafaring *Homo sapiens* followed a linear progression of dense kelp forests that lined the coast from Japan to Alaska to the southern point of California and then resumed along the Andean Coast from Peru to Tierra del Fuego.

Kelp forests are known to support complex food webs in coastal ecosystems. Such ecosystems are relatively homogenous and would have made it easier for migrating peoples to adapt to new territory as long as they followed the coastline. Kelp, fish, and shellfish are familiar foods to both an Eskimo in Alaska and an American Indian on the coast of Peru.

In a land migration, on the other hand, people would have encountered a variety of unfamiliar physical barriers and terrestrial ecosystems, from Arctic tundra to woodland forests, grasslands, and deserts. The animal and plant life varies widely in these landscapes, and it would have taken migrating people longer to figure out how to survive in their new environment. Erlandson also points out that some of the earliest settlements in North America are located adjacent to kelp forests, although the majority of the archaeological record of the kelp highway is most likely lost since ancient shorelines were buried under rising seas when the glaciers melted.

Homo sapiens already proved themselves to be expert navigators by this time, having been the only hominid species to reach Australia and other remote island groups roughly 50,000 years ago. Some of these islands were separated by over a hundred miles of open water, and yet there is evidence of early trade routes in the region, particularly for obsidian, the volcanic glass used to make stone tools (Harari 2015). The peopling of the Australian continent was even more impressive given the terrestrial life there was unlike anything *Homo sapiens* would have ever seen before. Giant marsupials dominated the landscape, from multi-ton wombats to 400-pound kangaroos and marsupial lions. Still, it is likely the earliest human visitors had little trouble finding something to eat. Kelp, fish, and shellfish are familiar foods to both an Eskimo in Alaska and a *Homo sapiens* on the coast of Australia.

In addition to Erlandson's Kelp Highway Hypothesis for explaining how *Homo sapiens* arrived in the Americas, anthropologists also use a coastal migration theory to explain the rapid expansion of *Homo sapiens* out of Africa, tracing a route to the Arabian Peninsula and then India, Southeast Asia, coastal China, Japan, New Guinea, Australia, and Oceania. Studies of genetics and linguistics support their theory. Even Weston Price on his visit to Africa commented on the similarity between the Ethiopians and the Polynesians he studied the previous year in the South Pacific, noting commonalities between certain words in their respective languages.

So here we are, on the shores of ancient Africa in our thinking backwards exercise. We traced the route of our *Homo sapiens* ancestors along a kelp highway from the mountains of Peru to the waters of the Pacific and then west to the birthplace of humanity. Surely this is where our hunt for milligram doses of iodine in the human diet must end, is it not?

The trail appears to go cold. Hominid predecessors in Africa were chimpanzees who evolved climbing trees and making funny banana jokes. They didn't eat seafood or drink milk. Their diet doesn't seem to hinge on the inclusion of eggs, blood, or organ meats. Archaeologists are *all kinds* of confused about how humanity happened, but they do have a theory on why early *Homo sapiens* decided to live at the beach.

During the second to last ice age, which started roughly 200,000 years ago, climate change in Africa turned rain forests and grasslands into desert. Some hominids like *Homo erectus* and *Homo neanderthalensis* had already made their way out of Africa by this time, but the hominids who would go on to become *Homo sapiens* remained on the continent where they were pushed to the brink of extinction. DNA analysis reveals lower than expected genetic variation in present-day humans, which anthropologists attribute to a dramatic population crash in early *Homo sapiens* (Marean 2010). It is possible the number of breeding individuals dwindled to a thousand or even fewer.

When Curtis Marean learned about the population bottleneck that geneticists were studying in the early 1990s, he was an archaeologist in East Africa's "cradle of humanity" studying the origin of modern humans. Marean began analyzing geologic formations, sea currents, and climate data to pinpoint a nondesertified region in Africa where early *Homo sapiens* could have survived the climatic upheaval caused by Marine Isotope Stage 6. His analysis led to the caves of South Africa where dropping ocean levels during the ice age would have revealed a slope of the continental shelf rich in marine life that washed in with the tides. In 1999, he identified a series of caves on a promontory that juts into the Indian Ocean as a promising place to start looking for evidence of early *Homo sapiens*. The spot is known as Pinnacle Point, and it proved to be hiding plenty of secrets Marean and his colleagues were about to uncover.

The excavations that followed unearthed a record of the *Homo sapiens* who lived along the coast of South Africa between 164,000 and 35,000 years ago, the time frame immediately after the bottleneck while the population was starting to recover. In 2007 Marean published his initial results in an article in *Nature* documenting that Pinnacle Point revealed the earliest known human use of marine resources and coastal habitats (Marean et al. 2007). *Homo sapiens* were consuming shellfish there as early as 164,000 years ago. This was a radical change from the terrestrial plants and animals that hominids were thought to have been consuming for millions of years.

But seafood was only the beginning of the revolutionary finds uncovered at Pinnacle Point. In 2009, Marean published another breakthrough in the journal *Science* demonstrating that heat-treated stone tools were already a dominant technology among *Homo sapiens* 71,000 years ago (Brown et al. 2009). Researchers previously believed the technology was invented in France just 20,000 years ago, but evidence from Pinnacle Point shows their conclusion was off by 50,000 years.

Early *Homo sapiens* in South Africa even used microlithic technology, small bladelets of heat-treated stones used to create advanced projectile weapons (Brown et al. 2012). The team also discovered dozens of pieces of red ochre at the site that showed signs they were ground into a powder and used as pigment. Marean argues this red ochre is the earliest unequivocal example of symbolic behavior. His research suggests that paleoanthropologists had been grossly underestimating the cognitive capabilities of early *Homo sapiens.*

The results of Marean's excavations at Pinnacle Point were published in a cover story in *Scientific American* entitled, "When the Sea Saved Humanity" (2010). In the article, Marean hypothesizes that *Homo sapiens* who migrated south to the sea during Marine Isotope Stage 6 thrived on the unique combination of plant and animal life in the famous Cape Floral Region of South Africa, an area that contains the highest diversity of flora for its size anywhere in the world. By studying the type of shells found in layers of sediment at the site, researchers were able to determine when the inhabitants figured out how to collect shellfish from deeper intertidal zones, indicating that 110,000 years ago, people scheduled their trips to the shore based on their observations of lunar effects on the tides.

In addition to shellfish, Marean also emphasizes the importance of geophytes in the early *Homo sapiens* diet. Geophytes are high-carbohydrate underground bulbs and tubers that Marean speculates early humans relied on as an easy source of dietary energy. His team did not uncover any evidence of geophyte consumption, however, which is not surprising since ancient organic matter is rarely preserved. Marean neglects to consider seaweed as an important factor in the evolution of modern humans, yet it is not difficult to imagine it being one of the first seafoods that *Homo sapiens* tasted. When humans first stepped onto the beach, why *wouldn't* they eat the edible plants the sea literally dropped at their feet with each new wave?

The story of modern humans is a story about returning to the sea. Prior to our exile from the African interior, early *Homo sapiens* were on the same evolutionary trajectory as other hominids. Our relatives from the genus *Homo* were an intelligent group. *Homo erectus* occupied Eurasia for well over a million years, making it the most enduring human species to ever walk the planet. Yet there is no indication they ever ventured to the shores of Australia. They were skilled hunters and are believed to be among the first hominids to use controlled fire, but their stone technology was relatively unchanged throughout their existence. *Homo sapiens* teenagers would never stand for that.

What made *Homo erectus* and *Homo sapiens* so different that one lived for nearly two million years as a relatively low-impact predator on the Eurasian landmass while the other exploded out of Africa roughly 100,000 years ago and quickly traveled to the farthest ends of the earth and beyond, altering everything in its path?

The experts speculate a variety of reasons for why *Homo sapiens* turned out to be such a dominant species—it is because we make complex tools, we learned how to hunt by throwing things, we trade food for sex, we're highly social.* But these explanations leave us largely unsatisfied because they are tautological. They are more a description of *how* humans behave rather than an explanation of *why* we came to behave this way.

The caves at Pinnacle Point are still being excavated and probably have many more secrets to tell, along with archaeological sites in the region yet to be discovered. But the most exciting find isn't the bits of shells and stones left at the site. Marean suggests that passing down complex processes from generation to generation—such as when to harvest food based on lunar observations, how to produce heat-treated weaponry, and how to create symbolic art—likely required the use of language.

---

*For several unsatisfying explanations and an equally unsatisfying explanation of why all the explanations are unsatisfying, see http://news.nationalgeographic.com/2015/09/150911 -how-we-became-human-theories-evolution-science

Language is not a uniquely human endeavor. Birds, dolphins, insects, monkeys, and all kinds of creatures use their own unique languages to communicate. But human language emerged to a complexity that enabled *Homo sapiens* to quickly jump to the top of the food chain and create civilizations, art, and technologies unlike anything that came before.

Linguists traditionally believed that human language gradually evolved from caveman grunts to the type of mumbling and pointing that goes on at the dentist's office and then eventually to the complex discussions we are capable of having today. But in recent studies, some linguists are challenging that gradualistic view (Nobrega and Miyazawa 2015). Instead, they believe human language arose very rapidly around 100,000 years ago from the integration of two preadapted systems— one from birdsongs and the other from the calls of nonhuman primates. Instead of a long, slow process when individual words were created and then strung together until sentences and paragraphs were born, Shigeru Miyazawa, a professor of linguistics at the Massachusetts Institute of Technology, explains that single words reveal traces of syntax showing they must be descended from an older, syntax-laden system. If Miyazawa is correct, then human language was created in one quick brush stroke of evolution.

Our search for milligram doses of iodine in the *Homo sapiens* diet ends here at the birthplace of human language roughly 100,000 years ago when our ancestors moved to the sea and began building the modern human civilization we are part of today. This convergence of events in the *Homo sapiens* story is not coincidental. Iodine has an undeniable effect on human cognition. The World Health Organization ranks a lack of dietary iodine as the single greatest cause of intellectual disability (de Benoist et al. 2008). Meanwhile, the Iodine Doctors report cases of their patients on iodine supplementation giving birth to children with IQ scores thirty points higher than either of their parents.*

---

*See Flechas's 2011 lecture entitled "Total Body Iodine Sufficiency" at www.HiddenCause ofAcne.com/Flechas

There is also an alarming body of research that shows fluoride—which inhibits iodine absorption—lowers IQ. The Fluoride Action Network identified fifty-six studies that investigate the relationship between fluoride and human intelligence.* Of those fifty-six studies, none of which were carried out in the United States, forty-nine found that fluoride exposure is associated with reduced intelligence, especially when combined with an iodine-deficient diet.†

In September 2017, a team of researchers funded by the National Institute of Health published the first study of fluoride's effect on IQ ever sponsored by the United States government. The results of the twelve-year study published in *Environmental Health Perspectives* identified a significant drop in intelligence for every 0.5 milligram-per-liter increase of fluoride exposure in utero (Bashash et al. 2017).

When researchers from Harvard conducted a meta-analysis of the literature, they concluded that the evidence was too great to ignore and that fluoride's neurotoxic effect on the human brain should be a "high research priority" (Choi et al. 2012). Iodine should also be considered in those studies. When *Homo sapiens* were forced to live off the sea for tens of thousands of years, it set into motion a cascade of creativity that currently manifests as space stations, supercomputers, symphonies, and nation states. I, too, experienced the rush of creative linguistic energy that comes with iodine. All at once, I had to write this book. I had to tell you my thoughts and ideas. I had to develop my voice and then use it.‡

Other species of hominids who didn't spend millennia at the sea never evolved in this way. Neanderthals lived their 200,000-year existence in small bands of nuclear families. They did not create the complex tools, advanced symbolic art, trade networks, and intricate social structures that are characteristic of *Homo sapiens*. In 1998, an American geographer named Jerome Dobson published a

---

*For more information, see http://fluoridealert.org/studies/brain01
†For more information, see http://fluoridealert.org/studies/thyroid01
‡See www.HiddenCauseofAcne.com/voice

study explaining that Neanderthal sites in Europe are often located in known iodine-deficient regions and that their skeletal systems and other traits have more in common with modern-day cretins than modern-day humans. He points to their thickened bones and muscles, protruding brows, and high incidence of degenerative joint disease as evidence, as well as the strange angular pattern of wear on their front teeth, which he asserts was caused by a protruding tongue, another sign of congenital hypothyroidism.

Scientists have made similar observations regarding *Homo floresiensis,* the hobbitlike human who lived on the Indonesian island of Flores as recently as 12,000 years ago (Oxnard, Obendorf, and Kefford 2010).

Isotopic analysis of Neanderthal bones reveals a dietary signature of a top-level carnivore similar to that of a hyena. Studies show their carnivorous diet was consistent over time and throughout different regions of Europe (Richards and Trinkaus 2009). In contrast, analysis of early *Homo sapiens* bones from the same region indicates a more varied diet, particularly from fish and shellfish, even amongst *Homo sapiens* living inland. In the Upper Paleolithic era, around 50,000 to 10,000 years ago when *Homo sapiens* first populated Europe, marine shells are commonly found hundreds of miles from their sources and were known to be worn as ornamentation by *Homo sapiens* hunter-gatherers who lived more than 300 miles inland (Dobson 1998).

A paleo diet is well and good, but we really should specify which kind of paleolithic hominid we are trying to emulate when we calculate the iodine requirement for modern humans.

Homo sapiens weren't the first mammals to return to the sea. As they say, history has a habit of repeating itself. Ungulates are the grouping of mammals that includes horses, cows, pigs, giraffes, camels, deer, and rhinoceros. In the 1970s, researchers in Pakistan discovered archaeological remains that show a progression of extinct ungulates who made their way to the ocean 55 million years ago.* They now exist as relatives

---

*See https://en.wikipedia.org/wiki/Evolution_of_cetaceans

of an ancient type of hippopotamus. We call them cetaceans: whales, porpoises, and dolphins.

Like *Homo sapiens,* cetaceans developed sophisticated forms of language when they took to the sea. Their vocalizations are so intricate and alien to *Homo sapiens* ears that we have yet to decipher their secrets. Cetaceans are known to use tools, compose music, and demonstrate creativity, self-awareness, complex play, and empathy. Also like *Homo sapiens,* they created elaborate social networks and proliferated in their new environment, spreading into virtually every corner of the ocean where they have thrived for millions of years.

Homo sapiens and cetaceans evolved from different mammalian lineages, but we share a common path from sea to land and back to sea once again. Cetaceans grew flippers, blowholes, and fins while *Homo sapiens* sprouted oars, hulls, and fishing lines. Frogs and other amphibious creatures also live at this crossroads, although in a different way. It has long been known that iodine is the controlling factor that guides their metamorphosis from aquatic to terrestrial beings (Galton 1992).

Iodine is a guiding element for all vertebrates. Through her studies of dogs and other domesticated animals, evolutionary zoologist Susan Crockford (2002) from the University of Victoria in British Columbia argues that thyroid hormone creates the "rhythm of life" that delineates new species. Other forms of life rely on iodine as well, from simple marine invertebrates like sponges and corals to sea urchins and unicellular planktonic algae. Sebastiano Venturi (2011), an iodine researcher in Italy, attempts the grand task of explaining the pivotal role of iodine in the evolution of life on earth, beginning with cyanobacteria, a type of blue-green algae that evolved 3.5 billion years ago with the advent of photosynthesis. Venturi describes iodine as the "most ancient and powerful antioxidant" and the oldest defense mechanism against oxygen produced by some of the earliest living cells.

If there is credence to Venturi's theory, then the story of iodine is the story of life. It explains why iodine is especially important for females and why nature concentrates it in mother's milk, eggs, and placental blood. It also explains why the traditional *Homo sapiens* diet, rich in milligram doses of iodine, produced the most creative creature to ever walk the shores of planet Earth.

So that's how the thinking backwards exercise works.

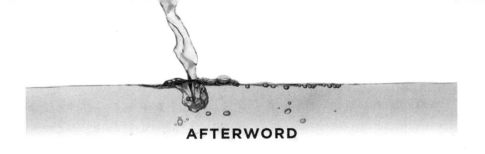

The End of Acne

Three things cannot be long hidden. The sun, the moon, and the truth.

BUDDHA

SO THERE YOU HAVE MY STORY of acne, my *anekdota*. Although I guess technically it's not an unpublished story anymore—presuming that if these words made their way to you it is because my story has been published.

I admit the idea of sending this book out into the world scares me a little. I just wrote a lot of words, and I'm sure some of them offended someone, some of them aren't as funny as I thought they were at the time, some of them are wrong, and some of them might spark discussions I don't want to be a part of. Intelligence analysts like myself value our quiet cubes and our anonymity. But there's too much going on in the world for me to stay in my cube. I'm done with it.

Your story of acne is the one that really matters. If the ideas I put forward in these pages don't resonate with your experience of the world, then I just wasted four months and all my vacation days writing a comic tragedy about raisins. Your story will decide the fate of mine. Will my ideas be crucified by the dental cult of fluoristanism? Whacked by dermatologist drug lords? Will they be the subject of a smear campaign by conniving mink oil manufacturers? And what will Dr. Oz and Cameron Diaz think of all this?

If this book doesn't help you heal your acne in a way that makes you want to tell other people about it, then my story about fluoride and acne ends here, and I will sink back into the shadows of my cubicle walls. But if these words changed your skin for the better, if you studied the ideas and the references and the footnotes and found them compelling, then our combined stories will shine a light on the myth that fluoride is safe and effective. And when the light comes on, we'll be ready for it.

This is not one of those books where I talk about something bad going on in our torn-up town and then give you obscure suggestions for little things you can do to help fix it. This is one of those books where we fix it. Together.

In the appendix that follows, you will see my seven-step plan to end fluoridation. Don't be deceived by its simplicity. As Leonardo da Vinci once said, simplicity is the ultimate sophistication. The first two steps of the plan will be completed by the time you read this, steps three to five are the most important (that's your part), and the last two steps will be crazy fun to do together. Notice each phase of the plan gets easier and none of them involve arguing with anyone or trying to change someone's mind.

Ending fluoridation will not be a fight and it's certainly not a war. It's more like breaking up with someone. In the dating world, when you realize a certain partner isn't right for you, we all know it is counterproductive to try to change them into who you want them to be, especially if they aren't eager to change. In this situation, it is best to move on. You'll need a recovery period, a time to find your footing (step one) and heal festering wounds (step two). It is healthy to talk with your friends about what went wrong in the relationship (step three), and if things were really bad, you might need to request a restraining order (step four) and find a support group to help you through it (step five). Before you know it, you will be back out on the town again living it up (step six) and looking to find someone new (step seven).

Growing up and growing old in this cynical *Homo sapiens* society our ancestors left us with, it is easy to become overwhelmed with all the negative stories that surround us. It is easy to feel small and power-less and to believe that things will never change. But that would be a sad analytic error to make. Change is the one thing we can count on. Change is constant and often unexpected. The experts continually change their minds even when they are the last to figure things out.

Fluoride *will* go the way of lead paint, asbestos, DDT, tobacco, and mercury-poisoned hatters. Someday psychologists will publish assessments in peer-reviewed journals of the twentieth-century fluoride craze. Pictures of a rare skin condition called acne will be included in textbooks for Health History 101, a required class for all *Homo sapiens* adolescents. After all these years struggling with acne, won't it be fun to be a part of that change?

The Smithsonian Institute didn't recognize the *Wright Flyer* as the first manned airplane until 1942. That didn't change the fact that the Wright brothers first flew it forty years prior. Smithsonian officials didn't want to embarrass their dead bureaucrats and tarnish the Institute's scientific reputation, but they were eventually forced to concede when a journalist threatened to write about the controversy in the Wright brothers' biography. What does this morsel of aviation history tell us? It tells us that the bureaucrats might have bigger voices than you and I do, but they are scared of us.

Promoters of fluoridation are scared too many of us will see through their story and then they will be forced to face the unthinkable: that their policies have been poisoning millions of people for generations. The current generation of dentists will likely never admit this, but that doesn't matter. Our goal is not to convince our ex to admit he's a jerk. Our goal is to end it and move on.

We don't need to convince everyone that fluoridation must end. Some people can't imagine questioning the current dental authorities, and most people won't care about it at all. We just need to reach the tipping point, which researchers estimate is between 15 and 18 percent market penetration. Fluoride activists like the Fluoride Action Network, Joseph Mercola, Erin Brockovich, and others are already working to reach that magic number. Celebrities like Alicia Silverstone, Suzanne Somers, Tom Brady, Martin Sheen, Ed Begley Jr., and Dr. Oz have been vocal about why they do not want fluoride in their drinking water.* When enough of us add our voices to theirs, the tipping point will be breached. The fluoridation myth will crack and then shatter, leaving nothing but shards beneath our feet.

Learning how to talk about fluoride in an intelligent, confident way is a critical step in the plan. In the past, I was embarrassed to tell people about my "fluoride allergy," but experience has shown that once I explain more of the details, most people see right through the lies bureaucrats tell. In my casual conversations with friends, family members, and coworkers about fluoride, I've found that there is one little-known secret that easily conveys the rest of the story: the fact that the fluoride added to the public water supply is gathered directly from the smokestacks of the phosphate fertilizer industry. For those of us who aren't caught up in their love affair with fluoride, this one fact is an ominous sign that fluoridation is a bad idea.

When you tell people that the fluoride in their drinking water is a toxic industrial waste product that Erin Brockovich herself came out swinging against, they will know fluoride isn't a story about children's sparkling white teeth.† They will know it's a pollution story. They will know the players. They will know the game. And they will know this is the start of how it all ends.

---

*Dr. Oz invited Erin Brockovich on his show to discuss public water fluoridation in a segment that aired February 1, 2016 (season 7, episode 89). On the webpage for the episode, instead of including a clip of the segment as is customary, Dr. Oz's team posted a disclaimer that his show should not be construed as medical advice alongside statements on the benefits of public water fluoridation from the Center for Disease Control, the American Dental Association, the American Association of Public Health Dentistry, the American Dental Hygienists' Association, and the Harvard School of Dental Medicine. There is no mention of Brockovich's appearance except for her name listed as a guest. To view the webpage for the episode in question, visit http://www.doctoroz .com/episode/breaking-news-zika-virus-public-health-emergency-making
†To read Erin Brockovich's statement on fluoride, see www.HiddenCauseofAcne.com/Erin

Here's why the way things change is about to change. We tell ourselves science is king, but our understanding of the world is shaped
through story. Historians have a theory that the way society is struc-
tured is a reflection of the primary means of communication. Since the
advent of human language, the storytellers have wielded disproportion-
ate influence over everyone else. When we abandoned oral tradition for
written myths that only a few powerful people could code and decode,
our communities grew and became more hierarchical and dogmatic.
Then with the printing press and the rise of literacy, we saw the birth
of democracy. Television and radio ushered in corporate fairy tales in
the guise of cartoon tigers and commercial breaks.

Looking back over recorded history, we can see the primary means
of storytelling has been largely one-sided. Someone with a megaphone
speaks, drowning out the rest of us. Our top-down societies are a reflection of this type of communication. The government issues a guideline
about how much fluoride your town should add to the water supply or
how much iodine your doctor should recommend for your diet, and we
have little choice but to listen. We can reject their guidelines on an individual level, but when we try to talk back, our tiny voices are virtually
incapable of being heard.

But peer-reviewed journal articles, books from elitist publishers,
and expensive network television and radio airtime are no longer our
society's primary means of storytelling. Nothing like Internet has ever
existed. Now the dentists post their story online, then I tell a story about
their story in an ebook, and then other people tell their stories about
my story about the dentists' story in the review section on Amazon.
People won't read my story unless your story indicates it's worth their
time. That is power. Now we're in the ring.

Sharing information is only a fraction of Internet's potential. In
1977 the United States held a congressional hearing on the science
of fluoridation after reports surfaced of a greater incidence of cancer
deaths in fluoridated communities. Congress ordered the U.S. Public
Health Service to have an independent contractor, Battelle Laboratory,

conduct animal studies to determine if fluoride is a carcinogen. The American public continued to consume fluoride while the studies were being conducted even though the final report took thirteen years to produce.

When the study was finally released, the controversial findings were the reason William Marcus, a toxicologist at the EPA's Office of Drinking Water, was fired in 1992 after he raised concerns that the results show fluoride causes cancer. After a two-year legal battle, a judge ordered that Marcus be reinstated under the Whistleblower Protection Act, but his concerns over the carcinogenicity of fluoride were never addressed.

In June 2000, Bill Hirzy, vice president of the EPA union of professional employees, testified on behalf of the union before the United States Senate to call for a moratorium on fluoridation until the evidence that fluoride causes cancer could be independently evaluated.* The moratorium never happened and neither did the cancer review. This will not do.

Internet was still a kid when all this happened, and so was I, but we've both done a lot of growing up since then. Together, you and I have the power to change things the way we want things to change. We can crack the code, and Internet is the trusty sidekick who will help us do it.

On December 2, 2015, the U.S. National Toxicology Program (NTP) held a hearing on the studies that indicate fluoride is a neurotoxin. They agreed the effects of fluoride on the developing brain are a "medium-to-high priority" and made plans to move forward with further research in the years ahead. If the U.S. National Toxicology Program is investigating fluoride as a neurotoxin, wouldn't it be wise for the U.S. Department of Health and Human Services to stop advising local governments to add it to drinking water? Seems like a reasonable request, right? Here's your chance to ask it to the people who can make it happen.

---

*To view Hirzy's presentation to Congress, see www.HiddenCauseofAcne.com/Hirzy

I set up a petition at Change.org to tell the U.S. government to stop recommending the addition of fluoride to public water supplies. Each time someone signs the petition, it will be delivered to the members of the Senate Subcommittee on Wildlife, Fisheries, and Drinking Water— the same committee Bill Hirzy testified in front of over fifteen years ago. It might take some time to gain momentum because our voices are dispersed and therefore difficult to make out, but if we focus them on one point in the internet ether we will eventually hear their true volume like an orchestra coming into tune. At that moment, I suspect we will realize we are bigger than we ever dreamed.

The story of how fluoridation ends is just beginning. You can help write it, two powerful words at a time.

Please add your name *right now*
to the petition to end fluoridation at
www.HiddenCauseofAcne.com/STOP.

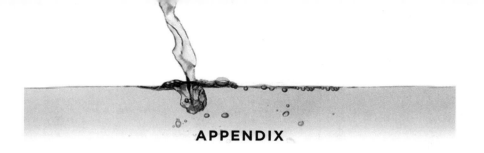

APPENDIX

The Plan

Step 1. ~~Write a book to tell people about fluoride and acne~~—*Me*

Step 2. ~~Create a website to help people with acne~~—*Me*

www.HiddenCauseofAcne.com/resources

www.HiddenCauseofAcne.com/guides

(go here for the cheat sheets)

Step 3. Help spread the word about fluoride and acne—*You*

- review *The Hidden Cause of Acne* on Amazon and Goodreads
- send your success stories to Melissa@ProjectFree.Me
- tweet your before and after pics (or just the after pics!) using #hiddencauseofacne (I'm @MelissaGallico)
- share your success story on Instagram or Tumblr using #hiddencauseofacne (I'm @MelissaGallico)

*Please do this one!

Step 4. Tell the United States federal government to stop recommending the addition of fluoride to public water supplies—*Us*

www.HiddenCauseofAcne.com/STOP

(click on the link to be redirected to the petition at Change.org)

Step 5. To make sure Congress follows through, join my email group—*You*

www.HiddenCauseofAcne.com/email

Step 6. Party like pop stars when we end fluoridation!—*Us*

(preferably in person, location TBD)

Step 7. Decide what part of this torn-up town we will fix next—*Us*

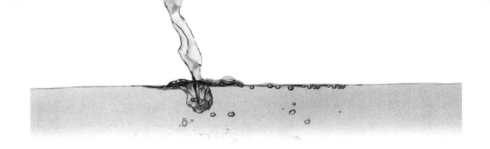

Acknowledgments

If you wish to make an apple pie from scratch, you must first invent the universe.

CARL SAGAN

I MIGHT HAVE BAKED A PIE, but I literally have a universe of people to thank for growing the apples, building the stove, and driving me to the bake sale. These are just a few of them.

Thank you to the good people at Google who lay a universe of information at the feet of my curious mind. Wikipedia, same. Thank you to the Fluoride Action Network for posting insane amounts of information about fluoride online. I never could have figured out how to heal my acne without it. Thank you to the Iodine Doctors and others like them who put their reputations and careers on the line every day for their patients by questioning the established health dogma. Thank you to Amazon for connecting me with the books and products I needed to put my theories to the test, and then for creating a home for my book when the time came to write about it all. Thank you to Apple for giving me the tools I needed to gather all that information and assemble it into a finished product. I will love you forever or until something better comes along. You know how it goes.

To the entire team at Inner Traditions, including the designers, the production team, Jon Graham, Kelly Bowen, Patricia Rydle, Manzanita Carpenter, Erica Robinson, Ashley Kolesnik, Jeanie Levitan, Elizabeth Wilson, and especially my smart and kindhearted project editor

Kayla Toher, thank you for your diligent work on this book, for taking a chance on a first-time author, and for being so nice.

To Stephen Harrod Buhner, thank you for teaching me how to follow a golden thread. I yanked that thread until the whole story unraveled and then used it to sew a sparkly gold dress. I am honored and humbled each time I look at your name on the cover next to mine. Thank you for believing in my work and for everything you did to help it find a wider audience.

Thank you to Hardy Limeback for your encouragement and support. Someday I will tell the story of the first time you emailed me, and people won't believe it. Thanks to Bill Hirzy and several of my analyst colleagues (you know who you are) for reading my entire 8,500-word exposé on raisins and providing constructive criticism. To my blogging buddy and eventual beta reader, Elizabeth Walling of The Nourished Life, thank you for reading an early copy of the manuscript for *The End of Acne* and providing valuable feedback.

To my original editor, Darlene Musso, thank you for conspiring with me on this project, for sharing your candid thoughts and ideas, for loving me like I grew up as part of the family, and for the perfect Christmas card you sent before you even knew I was writing a book about Inuits and cetaceans and language and the ocean. It hung above my writing desk and inspired me every day.* In case anyone was in doubt, this is hard proof you are an angel.

Thank you to my parents for telling me when I was a little girl (before I was old enough to mistake truth for cliché) that I can do anything I set my mind to. Thanks for the happiness in your voice when I call you on the phone and you realize it's me on the other side of the line. For how excited I know you will be when I tell you I wrote a book. For thinking the world of me. For your endless love. For all that and more. Thank you. It worked.

To sweet Gia, who reminds me every day that *Homo sapiens* are not

---

*www.HiddenCauseofAcne.com/writing-inspiration

the only beings being. And to my Marco, thank you for feeding me while I wrote this book. And for listening to me talk about raisins. And for never getting tired (or at least pretending not to get tired) of listening to me talk about raisins. I always say you are my dream man. But in truth, I could not have dreamed of a man as perfect for me as you are.

Finally, to everyone past and future who reads my story and realizes it is their own. Your testimonials are the reason this book exists. Thank you for sharing them with me. Thank you for reading even to this very last word.

Please, let's not make this goodbye.
www.HiddenCauseofAcne.com/email

References

To further explore the references cited in this book, please visit

www.HiddenCauseofAcne.com/resources

for links to journal articles, video evidence, and other resource material.

Abraham, Guy E. 2004. "The Safe and Effective Implementation of Orthoido-supplementation in Medical Practice." *The Original Internist* 11:17–36. http://www.optimox.com/iodine-study-5

———. 2005a. "The Historical Background of the Iodine Project." *The Original Internist* 12 (2): 57–66. http://www.optimox.com/iodine-study-8

———. 2005b. "The Wolff-Chaikoff Effect: Crying Wolf?" *The Original Internist* 12 (3): 112–18. http://www.optimox.com/iodine-study-4

———. 2006. "The History of Iodine in Medicine Part III: Thyroid Fixation and Medical Iodophobia." *The Original Internist* 13:71–78. http://www.optimox.com/iodine-study-16

Abraham, Guy E., J. D. Flechas, and J. C. Hakala. 2002. "Optimum Levels of Iodine for Greatest Mental and Physical Health." *The Original Internist* 9:5–20. http://www.optimox.com/iodine-study-1

Adebamowo, Clement, Donna Spiegelman, Catherine S. Berkey, F. William Danby, Helaine R. H. Rockette, Graham A. Colditz, Walter C. Willett, and Michelle D. Holmes. 2006. "Milk Consumption and Acne in Adolescent Girls." *Dermatology Online Journal* 12 (4): 1.

———. 2008. "Milk Consumption and Acne in Teenaged Boys." *Journal of the American Academy of Dermatology* 58 (5): 787–93.

Adebamowo, Clement, Donna Spiegelman, William Danby, A. Lindsay Frazier, Walter C. Willett, and Michelle D. Holmes. 2005. "High School Dietary Dairy Intake and Teenage Acne." *Journal of the American Academy of Dermatology* 52 (2): 207–14.

Adrasi, E. Cs. Bélavári, Vekoslava Stibilj, M. Dermelj, and D. Gawlik. 2003. "Iodine Concentration in Different Human Brain Parts." *Analytical and Bioanalytical Chemistry* 378 (1): 129–33.

Albuquerque, Rachel, Marco Alexandre Rocha, Ediléia Bagatin, S. Tufik, and Monica Andersen. 2014. "Could Adult Female Acne Be Associated with Modern Life?" *Archives of Dermatological Research* 306:683–88.

Alliance for a Cavity Free Future. n.d. "Milk Fluoridation." Accessed February 17, 2017, http://www.allianceforacavityfreefuture.org/en/us/technologies /systemic-fluorides/milk-fluoridation#.Vkxw_YSmSNY

American Academy of Dermatology. n.d. "Acne (Stats and Facts)." Accessed October 8, 2017, https://www.aad.org/media/stats/conditions

American Academy of Dermatology. n.d. "Acne: Tips for Managing Acne." Accessed February 16, 2017, www.aad.org/dermatology-a-to-z /diseases-and-treatments/a---d/acne/tips

American Thyroid Association. 2013. "ATA Statement on the Potential Risks of Excess Iodine Ingestion and Exposure." June 5, 2013. www.thyroid.org/ata -statement-on-the-potential-risks-of-excess-iodine-ingestion-and-exposure

Anderson, P. C. 1971. "Foods as the Cause of Acne." *American Journal of Family Practitioners* 3 (3): 102–3.

Arnold, Francis, Jr., H. Trendley Dean, and John Knutson. 1953. "Effect of Fluoridated Public Water Supplies on Dental Caries Prevalence." *Public Health Report* 68 (2): 141–48. http://www.ncbi.nlm.nih.gov/pmc/articles /PMC2024166/?page=1

Arnold, Francis, Jr., H. Trendley Dean, Philip Jay and John Knutson. 1956. "Effect of Fluoridated Public Water Supplies on Dental Caries Prevalence." *Public Health Report* 71 (7): 652–58. http://www.ncbi.nlm.nih.gov/pmc /articles/PMC2031043/?page=1

Arnold, Hubert A., to Ernest Newbrun. May 28, 1980. In *The Case Against Fluoride*. Paul Connett, James Beck, and H. Spedding Micklem. 2010. White River Junction, Vt.: Chelsea Green Publishing.

Bailey, DeeVon, and Michael R. Thomsen. 1994. "An Initial Analysis of the Mink Oil Market: Preliminary Report to Morgan County, Utah." Utah State University. *Economic Research Institute Study Papers*. Paper 31. http://

digitalcommons.usu.edu/cgi/viewcontent.cgi?article=1030&context=eri

Barkvoll, P. 1990. "Plasma F Levels Following Intake of NaF in Combination with Sodium Lauryl Sulphate." *Journal of Dental Research* 69:827.

Bashash, Morteza, Deena Thomas, Howard Hu, et al. 2017. "Prenatal Fluoride Exposure and Cognitive Outcomes in Children at 4 and 6–12 Years of Age in Mexico." *Environmental Health Perspectives* 125 (9). https://ehp.niehs.nih.gov/ehp655

Beltrán, Eugenio, Laurie Barker, and Bruce Dye. 2010. "Prevalence and Severity of Dental Fluorosis in the United States, 1999–2004." *National Center for Health Statistics Data Brief*, no. 53. https://www.cdc.gov/nchs/data/databriefs/db53.pdf

Bernays, Edward L. 1928. *Propaganda*. New York: Horace Liveright.

———. 1965. *Biography of an Idea: Memoirs of Public Relations Counsel*. New York: Simon and Schuster.

Bernays, Edward, to Leona Baumgartner, February 16, 1961. ELB papers, Baumgartner file. Library of Congress.

Bernecker, Christine. 1969. "Intermittent Therapy with Potassium Iodide in Chronic Obstructive Disease of the Airways." *Acta Allergologica* 24:216–25.

Bershad, Susan. 2003. "The Unwelcome Return of the Acne Diet." *Archives of Dermatology* 139 (7): 940–41. doi:10.1001/archderm.139.7.940-a.

Blasik, Lawrence, and Steven Spencer. 1979. "Fluoroderma." *Archives of Dermatology* 115 (11): 1334–35. doi: 10.1001/archderm.1979.04010110040022.

Blum, Arlene, Simona Balan, Martin Scheringer, Xenia Trier, Gretta Goldenman, Ian T. Cousins, Miriam Diamond, et al. 2015. "The Madrid Statement on Poly- and Perfluoroalkyl Substances (PFASs)." *Environmental Health Perspectives* 123 (5): A107–11. http://ehp.niehs.nih.gov/1509934

Response: Bowman, Jessica S. 2015. "Fluorotechnology Is Critical to Modern Life: The FluoroCouncil Counterpoint to the Madrid Statement." *Environmental Health Perspectives* 123 (5): A112–13. http://ehp.niehs.nih.gov/1509910

Reply to Bowman, Jessica, by Ian Cousins, Simona A. Balan, Martin Scheringer, Roland Weber, Zhanyun Wang, Arlene Blum, Miriam Diamond, et al. 2015. "Comment on 'Fluorotechnology Is Critical to Modern Life: The FluoroCouncil Counterpoint to the Madrid Statement.'" *Environmental Health Perspectives* 123 (7): A170. http://ehp.niehs.nih.gov/1510207

Jessica Bowman, 2015. "Response to 'Comment on "Fluorotechnology Is Critical to Modern Life: The FluoroCouncil Counterpoint to the Madrid

Statement,"'" *Environmental Health Perspectives* 123 (7): A170–71. http:// ehp.niehs.nih.gov/1510295

Blumenthal, Ralph. 2015. "New York's Fluoridation Fuss, 50 Years Later." *New York Times.* February 23, 2015. http://www.nytimes.com/2015/02/24 /health/new-yorks-fluoridation-fuss-50-years-later.html?_r=0

British Skin Foundation. 2015. "Over Half of Acne Sufferers Experience Verbal Abuse from Friends and Family Due to Their Condition." British Skin Foundation Press Release. http://www.britishskinfoundation.org.uk /LinkClick.aspx?fileticket=i2bE2n4c8m0%3D&tabid=172

Brown, Halina, Donna Bishop, and Carol Rowan. 1984. "The Role of Skin Absorption as a Route of Exposure for Volatile Organic Compounds (VOCs) in Drinking Water." *American Journal of Public Health* 74 (5): 479–84. https://www.ncbi.nlm.nih.gov/pmc/articles/PMC1651599/pdf /amjph00628-0063.pdf

Brown, Kyle S., Curtis W. Marean, Andy I. R. Herries, et al. 2009. "Fire as an Engineering Tool of Early Modern Humans." *Science* 325 (5942): 859–62.

Brown, Kyle S., Curtis W. Marean, Zenobia Jacobs, et al. 2012. "An Early and Enduring Advanced Technology Originating 71,000 Years Ago in South Africa." *Nature* 491:590–93.

Brown, Troy. 2015. "The 10 Most-Prescribed and Top-Selling Medications." Medscape Medical News. May 8, 2015. http://www.webmd.com/news /20150508/most-prescribed-top-selling-drugs

Brownstein, David. 2009. *Iodine: Why You Need It, Why You Can't Live Without It.* 4th ed. West Bloomfield, Mich.: Medical Alternatives Press.

Bryson, Christopher. 2011. *The Fluoride Deception.* New York: Seven Stories Press.

Bryun, G. W., and Charles M. Poser. 2003. *The History of Tropical Neurology: Nutritional Disorders.* Canton, Mass.: Science History Publications.

Burgstahler, A. W., and M. A. Robinson. 1997. "Fluoride in California Wines and Raisins." *Fluoride* 30 (3): 142–46.

California Department of Pesticide Regulation. 2013. "2013 County Summary Reports." Pesticide Use Reporting: 2013 Summary Data. www.cdpr.ca.gov /docs/pur/pur13rep/13_pur.htm

Camargo, Julio A. 2003. "Fluoride Toxicity to Aquatic Organisms: A Review." *Chemosphere* 50 (3): 251–64.

Camber, Rebecca. 2008. "Massive Increase in Dogs Poisoned by Chocolate and Grapes Fed to Them by Their Owners." *Daily Mail.* July 14, 2008.

http://www.dailymail.co.uk/news/article-1034677/Massive-increase-dogs
-poisoned-chocolate-grapes--fed-owners.html

Campaign for Safe Cosmetics. 2012. "Retailer Therapy." http://www.safecosmetics
.org/wp-content/uploads/2015/02/Retailer-Therapy-report.pdf

Cao, J., Y. Zhao, and J. Liu. 1997. "Brick Tea Consumption as the Cause of
Dental Fluorosis Among Children from Mongol, Kazak and Yugu populations in China." *Food and Chemical Toxicology* 35 (8): 827–33.

Carlsson, Arvid. 2005. "Water Fluoridation Obsolete According to Nobel Prize
Scientist." Interview by Michael Connett and Chris Neurath. Fluoride
Action Network, October 4, 2005. http://fluoridealert.org/content
/carlsson-interview

Center for Disease Control. 2015. "Private Wells." https://www.cdc.gov
/fluoridation/faqs/wellwater.htm

Chabris, Christopher, and Daniel Simons. 2009. *The Invisible Gorilla: How Our
Intuitions Deceive Us.* New York: Random House.

Chandrasekaran, Vali. 2011. "Correlation or Causation?" *Bloomberg Business.*
December 1, 2011. http://www.bloomberg.com/bw/magazine/correlation
-or-causation-12012011-gfx.html

Charlton, Rodger. 2000. "Value of Anecdotes." *Lancet* 355 (9212): 1372. http://
www.thelancet.com/journals/lancet/article/PIIS0140-6736(05)72613-1
/fulltext#back-bib2

Chikly, Bruno. 2001. *Silent Waves: Theory and Practice of Lymph Drainage
Therapy; With Applications for Lymphedema, Chronic Pain, and Inflammation.*
Palm Beach Gardens, Fl.: Upledger Institute.

Childers, Norman F., and M. D. Margoles. 1993. "An Apparent Relation
of Nightshades (Solanaceae) to Arthritis." *Journal of Neurological and
Orthopedic Medical Surgery* 12:227–31. http://noarthritis.com/research.htm

Choi, Anna L., Guifan Sun, Ying Zhang, and Philippe Grandjean. 2012.
"Developmental Fluoride Neurotoxicity: A Systematic Review and Meta-
Analysis." *Environmental Health Perspectives* 120 (10): 1362–68.

Cialdini, Robert. 1984. *Influence: The Psychology of Persuasion.* New York:
Harper Business.

Clark, Claudio. 1997. *Radium Girls, Women, and Industrial Health Reform:
1910-1935.* Chapel Hill: University of North Carolina Press.

Colquhoun, John. 1997. "Why I Changed My Mind about Water Fluoridation."
Perspectives in Biology and Medicine 41 (1): 29–44.

Connett, Michael. 2003. "The Phosphate Industry: An Environmental

Overview." Fluoride Action Network. http://fluoridealert.org/articles /phosphate01

———. 2012a. "Acute Fluoride Poisoning from Toothpaste Ingestion." Fluoride Action Network. http://fluoridealert.org/studies/acute03

———. 2012b. "Fluoridation, Dialysis & Osteomalacia." Fluoride Action Network. http://fluoridealert.org/studies/kidney04

———. 2012c. "Fluoride & Rheumatoid Arthritis." Fluoride Action Network. http://fluoridealert.org/studies/arthritis03

———. 2012d. "Hypersensitive Reactions to Topical Fluorides." Fluoride Action Network. http://fluoridealert.org/studies/hypersensitivity02

———. 2012e. "Skeletal Fluorosis in India and China." Fluoride Action Network. http://fluoridealert.org/studies/skeletal_fluorosis05

———. 2012f. "Tea Intake Is a Risk Factor for Skeletal Fluorosis." Fluoride Action Network. http://fluoridealert.org/studies/tea03

———. 2012g. "Tooth Decay Trends in Fluoridated vs. Unfluoridated Countries." Fluoride Action Network. http://fluoridealert.org/studies/caries01

———. 2015. "Fluoride Exposure Aggravates the Impact of Iodine Deficiency." http://fluoridealert.org/studies/thyroid01

Connett, Michael, and Tara Blank. 2016. "Fluoride and IQ: The 50 Studies." http://fluoridealert.org/studies/brain01

Connett, Paul, James Beck, and H. S. Micklem. 2010. *The Case Against Fluoride.* White River Junction, Vt.: Chelsea Green Publishing.

Cordain, Loren. 2006. *The Dietary Cure for Acne.* Fort Collins, Colo.: Paleo Diet Enterprises.

———. 2011. "Dr. Pastore's Questions." The Paleo Diet (blog). http://thepaleo diet.com/dr-pastores-qa-with-dr-cordain

———. 2015. "Exclusive Interview with Godfather of Paleo Loren Cordain!" Interview by Paleo Café, July 24, 2015. https://web.archive.org /web/20160714100033/http://paleo-cafe.com.au/2015/07/exclusive -interview-paleo-founder-loren-cordain

Cordain, Loren, Staffan Lindeberg, and Magdalena Hurtado. 2002. "Acne Vulgaris: A Disease of Western Civilization." *Archives of Dermatology* 138 (12): 1584–90. doi:10.1001/archderm.138.12.1584.

Cos, Theo, Abraham D. Flaxman, Mohsen Naghavi, et al. 2012. "Years Lived with Disability (YLDs) for 1160 Sequelae of 289 Diseases and Injuries 1990–2010: A Systematic Analysis for the Global Burden of Disease Study 2010." *Lancet* 380 (9859): 2163–96.

Crockford, Susan J. 2002. "Commentary: Thyroid Hormone in Neandertal Evolution: A Natural or a Pathological Role?" *Geographical Review* 92 (1): 73–88.

Curzon, M. E. J., and J. A. Curzon. 1979. "Dental Caries Prevalence in the Baffin Island Eskimo." *Pediatric Dentistry* 1 (3): 169–73. http://www.aapd.org/assets/1/25/Curzon-01-03.pdf

Dai, G., Z. Zhang, C. Qian, C. Zhai, and H. Gao. 2004. "Distributive Regulation of Bone Substance Change in Various Population Sub-groups with Different Fluoride Concentrations in Drinking Water." *Chinese Journal of Endemiology* 2004-02.

Danby, William F. 2007. "Acne and Iodine: Reply." *Journal of the American Academy of Dermatology* 56 (1): 164–65.

Dean, Trendley H., F. A. Arnold Jr., P. Jay, and J. W. Knutson. 1950. "Studies on Mass Control of Dental Caries through Fluoridation of the Public Water Supply." Public Health Report 65 (43): 1403–8. http://www.ncbi.nlm.nih.gov/pmc/articles/PMC1997106/?page=21

DeAngelo, Anthony B., Michael H. George, Steve R. Kilburn, Tanya M. Moore, and Douglas C. Wolf. 1998. "Carcinogenicity of Potassium Bromate Administered in the Drinking Water to Male B6C3F1 Mice and F344/N Rats." *Journal of Toxicologic Pathology* 26 (5): 587–94.

de Benoist, Bruno, Erin McLean, Maria Andersson, and Lisa Rogers. 2008. "Iodine Deficiency in 2007: Global Progress Since 2003." *Food and Nutrition Bulletin* 29 (3): 195–202. http://www.who.int/nutrition/publications/micronutrients/FNBvol29N3sep08.pdf?ua=1

Dennis, L. 1878. "Hatting: As Effecting the Health of Operatives." *Report of the New Jersey State Board of Health* 2:67–85, as quoted in R. P. Wedeen. 1989. "Were the Hatters of New Jersey 'Mad'?" *American Journal of Industrial Medicine* 16 (2): 225–33.

DeSimone, Leslie A., Pixie A. Hamilton, and Robert J. Gilliom. 2009. "Quality of Water from Domestic Wells in Principal Aquifers of the United States, 1991–2004." *U.S. Geological Survey Scientific Investigations Report* 2008–522. https://pubs.usgs.gov/sir/2008/5227/includes/sir2008-5227.pdf

Diaz, Cameron. 2013. *The Body Book.* New York: Harper Collins Publishers.

Dillehay, Tom D., C. Ramírez, M. Pino, M. B. Collins, J. Rossen, and J. D. Pino-Navarro. 2008. "Monte Verde: Seaweed, Food, Medicine, and the Peopling of South America." *Science* 320 (5877): 784–86. doi: 10.1126/science.1156533.

Diouf, A., F. O. Sy, B. Niane, D. Ba, and M. Ciss. 1994. "Dietary Intake of Fluorine through Use of Tea Prepared by the Traditional Method in Senegal." *Dakar Medical* 39 (2): 227–30.

Dobson, Jerome E. 1998. "The Iodine Factor in Health and Evolution." *Geographical Review* 88 (1): 3–28.

Downing, Donald, Anna Stranieri, and John Strauss. 1982. "The Effect of Accumulated Lipids on Measurements of Sebum Secretion in Human Skin." *Journal of Investigative Dermatology* 79 (4): 226–28.

Dreno, B. 2015. "Treatment of Adult Female Acne: A New Challenge." *Journal of the European Academy of Dermatology and Venereology* 29 (S5): 14–19.

Dreno, B., A. Layton, C. C. Zouboulis, et al. 2013. "Adult Female Acne: A New Paradigm." *Journal of the European Academy of Dermatology and Venereology* 27 (9): 1063–70.

Ekstrand, Joseph. 1987. "Pharmacokinetic Aspects of Topical Fluorides." *Journal of Dental Research* 66 (5): 1061–65.

Ekstrand, J., L. O. Boreus, and P. de Chateau. 1981. "No Evidence of Transfer of Fluoride from Plasma to Breast Milk." *British Medical Journal* (Clinical research ed.) 283 (6294): 761–62. http://www.ncbi.nlm.nih.gov/pmc/articles/PMC1506856/?page=1

Ekstrand, Joseph, and Goran Koch. 1980. "Systemic Fluoride Absorption Following Fluoride Gel Application." *Journal of Dental Research* 59 (6): 1067.

Elf Atochem North America, Inc. n.d. "Kryocide Advisory on Use of Cryolite to Control Insects on Grapes." Fluoride Action Network. Accessed February 17, 2017, http://fluoridealert.org/content/kryocide-advisory-grapes

Elsair, J., R. Merad, R. Denine, et al. 1981. "Boron as Antidote to Fluoride: Effect on Bones and Claws in Subacute Intoxication of Rabbits." *Fluoride* 14 (1): 21–29. http://www.fluorideresearch.org/141/files/FJ1981_v14_n1_p001-048.pdf

Elsair, J., R. Merad, R. Denine, et al. 1980. "Boron as an Antidote in Acute Fluoride Intoxication in Rabbits: Its Action on the Fluoride and Calcium-phosphorous Metabolism." *Fluoride* 13 (1): 30–38.

Environmental Protection Agency. 2002. "Sulfuryl Fluoride: Temporary Pesticide Tolerances." *Federal Register* 67 (26): 5735–5740. http://www.gpo.gov/fdsys/pkg/FR-2002-02-07/pdf/02-2983.pdf

———. 2011. "Cryolite Summary Document Registration Review: Initial Docket March 2011." http://www.regulations.gov/#!documentDetail;D=EPA-HQ-OPP-2011-0173-0008

Erlandson, Jon M., Michael H. Graham, Bruce J. Bourque, Debra Corbett, James A. Estes, and Robert S. Steneck. 2001. "The Kelp Highway Hypothesis: Marine Ecology, the Coastal Migration Theory, and the Peopling of the Americas." *Journal of Island and Coastal Archaeology* 2 (2): 161–74.

Eubig, Paul A., Melinda S. Brady, Sharon M. Gwaltney-Brant, Safdar A. Khan, Elisa M. Mazzaferro, and Carla M. K. Morrow. 2005. "Acute Renal Failure in Dogs After the Ingestion of Grapes or Raisins: A Retrospective Evaluation of 43 Dogs (1992–2002)." *Journal of Veterinary Internal Medicine* 19:663–74. http://onlinelibrary.wiley.com/doi/10.1111/j.1939-1676.2005.tb02744.x/epdf

Farrow, Lynne. 2013. *The Iodine Crisis: What You Don't Know About Iodine Can Wreck Your Life*. New York: Devon Press.

Fein, Noelle J., and Florian L. Cerklewski. 2001. "Fluoride Content of Foods Made with Mechanically Separated Chicken." *Journal of Agricultural and Food Chemistry* 49 (9): 4284–86.

Feltman, Reuben. 1956. "Prenatal and Postnatal Ingestion of Fluoride Salts: A progress report." *Dental Digest* 62: 353–57.

Feltman, Reuben, and George Kosel. 1961. "Prenatal and Postnatal Ingestion of Fluorides: Fourteen Years of Investigation; Final report." *Journal of Dental Medicine* 16:190–99.

Ferriss, Timothy. 2007. *The 4-Hour Workweek: Escape 9-5, Live Anywhere, and Join the New Rich*. New York: Crown Publishing Group.

"Five Controversial Food Additives." 2008. *Newsweek*. March 12, 2008. http://www.newsweek.com/five-controversial-food-additives-83551

Formella, Timothy M. 2002. "Petition for the listing of Cryolite on the USDA National List of Allowed and Prohibited Substances." Submitted by Cerexagri, Inc. to National Organic Standards Board on October 25, 2002. http://www.ams.usda.gov/sites/default/files/media/Cryolite%20Petition.pdf

Fraysse, C., M. W. Bilbeissi, D. Mitre, and B. Kerebl. 1989. "The Role of Tea Consumption in Dental Fluorosis in Jordan." *Bulletin du Groupement International pour la Recherche Scientifique en Stomatologie et Odontologie* 32 (1): 39–46. [Article in French]

Freeman, Addison J. 1860. "Mercurial Disease Among Hatters." *Transactions of the Medical Society of New Jersey*: 61–64, as quoted in "Erethism," Wikipedia. https://en.wikipedia.org/wiki/Erethism#References

Full, C. A., and Frederick Parkins. 1975. "Effect of Cooking Vessel Composition on Fluoride." *Journal of Dental Research* 54:192. http://jdr.sagepub.com /content/54/1/192.extract

Fulton, James, Gerd Plewig, and Albert Kligman. 1969. "Effect of Chocolate on Acne Vulgaris." *Journal of the American Medical Association* 210:2071–74. doi:10.1001/jama.1969.03160370055011.

Galletti, Pierre M., and Gustave Joyet. 1958. "Effect of Fluorine on Thyroidal Iodine Metabolism in Hyperthyroidism." *Journal of Clinical Endocrinology* 18:1102–10.

Galton, Valeria A. 1992. "The Role of Thyroid Hormone in Amphibian Metamorphosis." *Trends in Endocrinology & Metabolism* 3 (3): 96–100.

Ganim, Sara. 2015. "10-year-old hospitalized after termite fumigation." *CNN,* September 5. http://www.cnn.com/2015/09/04/us/termite-fumigation -hospitalization

Geek. 2004. "My Big Fat Greek Leukonychia." SalonGeek. July 12, 2004. http:// www.salongeek.com/threads/my-big-fat-greek-leukonychia.6245

Ghent, W. R., B. A. Eskin, D. A. Low, and L. P. Hill. 1993. "Iodine Replacement in Fibrocystic Disease of the Breast." *Canadian Journal of Surgery* 36:453–60.

Gillespie, George M., and Ramon Baez. 2005. "Development of Salt Fluoridation in the Americas." *Schweiz Monatsschr Zahnmed* 115:663–69. https:// www.sso.ch/fileadmin/upload_sso/2_Zahnaerzte/2_SDJ/SMfZ_2005 /SMfZ_08_2005/smfz-08-forschung-5.pdf

Gomez, S. Sergio, A. Weber, and C. Torres. 1989. "Fluoride Content of Tea and Amount Ingested by Children." *Odontologia Chilena* 37 (2): 251–55. [Article in Spanish]

Gotzfried, Franz. 2006. "Legal Aspects of Fluoride in Salt, Particularly Within the EU." *Schweiz Monatsschr Zahnmed* 116:371–75. http://www.fluoride- alert.org/wp-content/uploads/gotzfried-2006.pdf

Grant, Tara. 2013. *The Hidden Plague: A Field Guide for Surviving and Overcoming Hidradenitis Suppurativa.* Malibu, Calif.: Primal Blueprint Publishing.

Green, Emily. 2000. "Is Milk Still Milk?" *Los Angeles Times,* August 2, 2000. http://articles.latimes.com/2000/aug/02/food/fo-62752

Greene, Jeff. 2012. "Non-Organic Foods Blast Your Body with Up to 180 Times the Fluoride in Drinking Water." Interview by Joseph Mercola, February 4, 2012. http://articles.mercola.com/sites/articles/archive/2012/02/04/jeff -green-on-fluoride-toxins-part-2.aspx

Greene, Robert. 2012. *Mastery.* New York: The Penguin Group.

Greep, Roy O., and Monte A. Greer. 1985. *Edwin Bennett Astwood, 1909–1976: A Biographical Memoir*. Washington, D.C.: National Academy of Sciences. http://www.nasonline.org/publications/biographical-memoirs/memoir-pdfs/astwood-edwin-b.pdf

Gupta, M. A., and Aditya Gupta. 1998. "Depression and Suicidal Ideation in Dermatology Patients with Acne, Alopecia Areata, Atopic Dermatitis and Psoriasis." *British Journal of Dermatology* 139:846–50.

Guyenet, Stephan. 2009. Comments on "Iodine." Whole Health Source (blog). http://wholehealthsource.blogspot.com/2009/05/iodine.html

Hampl, Jeffrey, and William Hampl. 1997. "Pellagra and the Origin of a Myth: Evidence from European Literature and Folklore." *Journal of the Royal Society of Medicine* 90 (11): 636–39. http://www.ncbi.nlm.nih.gov/pmc/articles/PMC1296679/?page=1

Hanlon, Patrick. 2006. *Primal Branding: Create Zealots for Your Brand, Your Company, and Your Future*. New York: Free Press.

Harari, Yuval Noah. 2015. *Sapiens: A Brief History of Humankind*. New York: HarperCollins Publishers.

Harvard Health Publishing. 2011. "When Depression Starts in the Neck." Harvard Mental Health Letter. http://www.health.harvard.edu/newsletter_article/when-depression-starts-in-the-neck

Health Canada. 1993. "Inorganic Fluorides: Priority Substances List Assessment Report." http://www.hc-sc.gc.ca/ewh-semt/pubs/contaminants/psl1-lsp1/fluorides_inorg_fluorures/index-eng.php

Heilman, Judy R., Mary C. Kirtsy, Steven M. Levy, and James S. Wefel. 1999. "Assessing Fluoride Levels of Carbonated Soft Drinks." *Journal of the American Dental Association* 130 (11): 1593–99.

Heuer, Richards J., Jr. 2013. *Psychology of Intelligence Analysis*. Washington, D.C.: Center for the Study of Analysis. https://www.cia.gov/library/center-for-the-study-of-intelligence/csi-publications/books-and-monographs/psychology-of-intelligence-analysis/

Hirzy, William. 2000. "Why EPA's Headquarters Professionals' Union Opposes Fluoridation." Fluoride Action Network. http://fluoridealert.org/articles/epa-union

Hitch, Joseph M., and Bernard G. Greenburg. 1961. "Adolescent Acne and Dietary Iodine." *Archives of Dermatology* 84 (6): 898–911.

Jackson, Robert. 1974. "Non-bacterial Pus-forming Diseases of the Skin." *Canadian Medical Association Journal* 111 (8): 801, 804–06.

Jeans, P. C. 1953. "A Survey of the Literature of Dental Caries Prepared for the National Research Council." *Science* 117 (3042): 436–37. doi: 10.1126 /science.117.3042.436-a.

John, Finn J. D. 2012. "Horrifying Asylum Kitchen Mix-up Left Dozens Dead." *Offbeat OREGON,* November 19, 2012. http://offbeatoregon.com/1211c -asylum-kitchen-mixup-killed-hundreds-with-scrambled-eggs.html

Kahneman, Daniel. 2011. *Thinking Fast and Slow.* New York: Farrar, Straus and Giroux.

Kay, Jane. 2014. "Banned Scotchgard Chemical Still Contaminating San Francisco Seals." *Environmental Health News,* January 30, 2014. http:// www.environmentalhealthnews.org/ehs/news/2014/jan/bay-seals-and-pfos

Kearns, Cristin, Stanton A. Glantz, and Laura Schmidt. 2015. "Sugar Industry Influence on the Scientific Agenda of the National Institute of Dental Research's 1971 National Caries Program: A Historical Analysis of Internal Documents." *PLoS Medicin*e 12 (3): e100179. doi:10.1371/journal .pmed.1001798.

Kiritsy, Mary C., Steven M. Levy, John J. Warren, Nupurguha-Chowdhury, Judy R. Heilman, and Teresa Marshall. 1996. "Assessing Fluoride Concentrations of Juices and Juice-flavored Drinks." *Journal of the American Dental Association* 127 (7): 895–902.

Kitzmiller, Kathryn J. n.d. "The Not-So-Mad Hatter: Occupational Hazards of Mercury." *Science Connections.* Chemical Abstracts Service. Accessed February 17, 2017, https://www.cas.org/news/insights/science-connections /mad-hatter

Kuhnlein, Harriet V., and Nancy K. Turner. 1991. *Traditional Plant Foods of Canadian Indigenous Peoples: Nutrition, Botany and Use.* Food and Agriculture Organization of the United Nations: Agriculture and Consumer Protection Department. Amsterdam: Overseas Publishers Association. http://www.fao.org/wairdocs/other/ai215e/ai215e06.htm

Lamberg, Matti, Hannu Hausen, and Terttu Vartiainen. 1997. "Symptoms Experienced During Periods of Actual and Supposed Water Fluoridation." *Community Dentistry and Oral Epidemiology* 25 (4): 291–95.

Lehava, Noah. n.d. "Olivia Munn Swears Cutting Fluoride Cleared Her Acne." Coveteur. Accessed September 21, 2017, http://coveteur.com/2017/06/29 /olivia-munn-beauty-routine-cutting-fluoride-cleared-acne

Lehmann, Harold, Karen A. Robinson, John S. Andrews, Victoria Holloway, and Steven M. Goodman. 2002. "Acne Therapy: A Methodologic Review."

Journal of the American Academy of Dermatology 47:231–40. doi: http://dx.doi.org/10.1067/mjd.2002.120912

Leung, Angela M., Lewis E. Braverman, and Elizabeth N. Pearce. 2012. "History of U.S. Iodine Fortification and Supplementation." *Nutrients* 4 (11): 1740–46.

Li, Chinlei, Xiao Yang, Jianhui Hu, and Dejiang Ni. 2013. "Effect of Fluoride on Aroma of Tea Leaves." *Fluoride* 46 (1): 25–28. http://www.fluoride research.org/461/files/FJ2013_v46_n1_p025-028_sfs.pdf

Limeback, Hardy. 2000. "Why I Am Now Officially Opposed to Adding Fluoride to Drinking Water." Fluoride Action Network. http://fluoride alert.org/articles/limeback

Linton, Ron. 1970. *Terracide: America's Destruction of Her Living Environment.* New York: Little Brown & Company.

London, William T., R. L. Vought, and Freddie A. Brown. 1965. "Bread: A Dietary Source of Large Quantities of Iodine." *New England Journal of Medicine* 273 (7): 273–381.

Luke, Jennifer. 1997. "The Effect of Fluoride on the Physiology of the Pineal Gland." Ph.D. diss. University of Surrey. http://fluoridealert.org/studies /luke-1997

Lute, Rubén J., Miguel Fridmanis, Alejandro L. Misiunas, et al. 1985. "Association of Melasma with Thyroid Autoimmunity and other Thyroidal Abnormalities and Their Relationship to the Origin of the Melasma." *Journal of Clinical Endocrinology and Metabolism* 61 (1): 28–31.

Machaliński, B. 1996. "Concentration and Distribution of Fluorine in Hen's Eggs as an Aspect of Selected Biological Parameters." *Annales Academiae Medicae Stetinensis* 42:25–38. [Article in Polish]

Mahadevan, T. N., V. Meenaksy, and U. C. Mishra. 1986. "Fluoride Cycling in Nature through Precipitation." *Atmospheric Environment* 20 (9): 1745–49.

Mahvi, Amir Hossein, Maryam Ghanbarian, Marjan Ghanbarian, Ahmad Khosravi, and Masoud Ghanbarian. 2012. "Determination of Fluoride Concentration in Powdered Milk in Iran 2010." *British Journal of Nutrition* 107 (7): 1077–79.

Main, Douglas. 2015a. "Fluoridation May Not Prevent Cavities, Scientific Review Shows." *Newsweek,* June 29, 2015. http://www.newsweek.com /fluoridation-may-not-prevent-cavities-huge-study-shows-348251

———. 2015b. "Water Fluoridation Linked to Higher ADHD Rates."

Newsweek, March 10, 2015. http://www.newsweek.com/water-fluoridation
-linked-higher-adhd-rates-312748

Malin, Ashley, and Christine Till. 2015. "Exposure to Fluoridated Water and
Attention Deficit Hyperactivity Disorder Prevalence among Children
and Adolescents in the United States: An Ecological Association."
Environmental Health 14:17.

Marcovitch, S., and W. W. Stanley. 1942. "A Study of Antidotes for Fluorine."
Journal of Pharmacology and Experimental Therapeutic 74 (2): 235–38.

Marcus, William. 1995. "Interview with EPA's Dr. William Marcus on NTP's
Fluoride/Cancer Study." Interview by Gary Null. Fluoride Action Network.
Transcript #310. http://fluoridealert.org/content/marcus-interview

Marean, Curtis W. 2010. "When the Sea Saved Humanity." *Scientific American,*
August 2010.

Marean, Curtis W., Miryam Bar-Matthews, Jocelyn Bernatchez, et al. 2007.
"Early Human Use of Marine Resources and Pigment in South Africa
During the Middle Pleistocene." *Nature* 449:905–8.

Marinho, Valerie, Dominic Hurst, Ramon Baez, and Thomas M. Marthaler.
2016. "Salt Fluoridation for Preventing Dental Caries." *Cochrane Database
of Systematic Reviews,* May 10, 2016. http://onlinelibrary.wiley.com
/doi/10.1002/14651858.CD006846.pub2/abstract

Marinho, V.C.C., H. V. Worthington, T. Walsh, and L. Chong. 2015. "Fluoride
Gels for Preventing Dental Caries in Children and Adolescents." *Cochrane
Database of Systematic Reviews,* June 15, 2015. http://www.cochrane.org
/CD002280/ORAL_fluoride-gels-for-preventing-tooth-decay-in-children
-and-adolescents

Marthaler, Thomas M. 2005. "Overview of Salt Fluoridation in Switzerland
Since 1955, A Short History." *Schweiz Monatsschr Zahnmed* 115:651–55.
https://www.sso.ch/fileadmin/upload_sso/2_Zahnaerzte/2_SDJ
/SMfZ_2005/SMfZ_08_2005/smfz-08-forschung-2.pdf

Maslin Nir, Sarah. 2015. "Perfect Nails, Poisoned Workers." *New York Times,*
May 8, 2015. http://www.nytimes.com/2015/05/11/nyregion/nail-salon
-workers-in-nyc-face-hazardous-chemicals.html?_r=0)

McDonough, John, and Karen Egolf, eds. 2002. *The Advertising Age:
Encyclopedia of Advertising.* Chicago: Fitzroy Dearborn Publishers.

McFadden, Robert D. 1979. "$750,000 Given in Child's Death in Fluoride
Case." *New York Times,* January 20, 1979. http://fluoridealert.org/articles
/kennerly

Means, Charlotte. 2002. "The Wrath of Grapes." *ASPCA Animal Watch 22.* http://web.archive.org/web/20090205172006/http://www.aspca.org/site /DocServer/grapes.pdf?docID=189

Medical College of Georgia. 2010. "Tea Contains More Fluoride Than Once Thought." Public release from the Medical College of Georgia, Georgia Regents University, July 14, 2010. http://www.eurekalert.org/pub _releases/2010-07/mcog-tcm071410.php

Mullenix, Phyllis. 2000. "Fluoride & the Brain: An Interview with Dr. Phyllis Mullenix." Interview by Paul Connett. Fluoride Action Network, October 18, 1997. http://fluoridealert.org/content/mullenix-interview/

Mullenix, Phyllis, P. K. Denbesten, A. Schunior, and W. J. Kernan. 1995. "Neurotoxicity of Sodium Fluoride in Rats." *Neurotoxicology and Teratology* 17 (2): 169–77.

National Research Council. 1952. *A Survey of the Literature of Dental Caries.* Washington, D.C.: National Academies Press. https://doi.org/10.17226 /21295

National Research Council of the National Academies. 2006. "Fluoride in Drinking Water: A Scientific Review of EPA's Standards." http://www.nap. edu/read/11571

Nierenberg, Andrew A., Maurizio Fava, Madhukar H. Trivedi, et al. 2006. "A Comparison of Lithium and T 3 Augmentation Following Two Failed Medication Treatments for Depression: A STAR*D Report." *American Journal of Psychiatry* 163 (9): 1519–30. http://ajp.psychiatryonline.org/doi /full/10.1176/ajp.2006.163.9.1519

"No Worries about Cryolite Here." 2007. *Seattle Times,* January 17, 2007. http://www.seattletimes.com/food-drink/no-worries-about-cryolite-ere

Nobrega, Vitor A., and Shigeru Miyazawa. 2015. "The Precedence of Syntax in the Rapid Emergence of Human Language in Evolution as Defined by the Integration Hypothesis." *Frontiers in Psychology* 6:271.

Oaklander, Mandy. 2014. "The New Science of Clear Skin." *Prevention.* http:// www.prevention.com/beauty/natural-beauty/new-science-clear-skin

Olney, Richard S., Scott D. Grosse, and Robert F. Vogt Jr. 2010. "Prevalence of Congenital Hypothyroidism—Current Trends and Future Directions: Workshop Summary." *Pediatrics* 125 (2): 31–36. http://pediatrics.aap publications.org/content/125/Supplement_2/S31.full

Oxnard, Charles, Peter J. Obendorf, and Ben K. Kefford. 2010. "Post-Cranial Skeletons of Hypothyroid Cretins Show a Similar Anatomical Mosaic as

Homo floresiensis." *PLoS ONE* 5 (9): e13018. https://doi.org/10.1371/journal .pone.0013018

Oz, Mehmet. 2012. "My Father-in-Law's Best Health Advice." The Oz Blog, November 19, 2012. http://blog.doctoroz.com/dr-oz-blog /my-father-in-laws-best-advice

Oz, Mehmet C., and Michael F. Roizen. 2005. *YOU: The Owner's Manual: An Insider's Guide to the Body That Will Make You Younger and Healthier.* New York: Collins Publishers.

Perkins, Alexis C., Jessica Maglione, Greg G. Hillebrand, Kukizo Miyamoto, and Alexa B. Kimball. 2012. "Acne Vulgaris in Women: Prevalence Across the Life Span." *Journal of Women's Health* 21 (2): 223–23.

Petersen, P. E., and Prathip Phantumvanit. 2012. "Toward Effective Use of Fluoride in Asia." *Advances in Dental Research* 24 (1): 2–4. http://adr.sage pub.com/content/24/1/2

Physicians' Desk Reference, 1994, 48th ed. Montvale, NJ: Medical Economics Data Production Co. As cited in "Physician's Desk Reference: Fluoride Hypersensitivity." n.d. Fluoride Action Network. Accessed February 15, 2017, http://fluoridealert.org/studies/hypersensitivity03

Pradhan, K. M., N. K. Arora, A. Jena, S. K. Andezhath, and M. K. Bhan. 1995. "Safety of Ciprofloxacin Therapy in Children: Magnetic Resonance Images, Body Fluid Levels of Fluoride and Linear Growth." *Acta Paediatrica* 84 (5): 555–60.

Price, Weston A. 1935. "Studies of Relationships Between Nutritional Deficiencies and (a) Facial and Dental Arch Deformities and (b) Loss of Immunity to Dental Caries Among South Sea Islanders and Florida Indians." *Dental Cosmos* 77 (11): 1033–45.

———. 1939. *Nutrition and Physical Degeneration*. New York: Harper & Brothers.

Prival, Michael. 1972. *Fluorides and Human Health*. Washington, D. C.: Center for Science in the Public Interest.

Ramsey Mellette, J., John Aeling, and Donald Nuss. 1983. "Perioral Dermatitis." *Journal of the Association of Military Dermatologists* 9:3–8. http://fluoride alert.org/studies/mellette-1983

Richards, Michael P., and Erik Trinkaus. 2009. "Isotopic Evidence for the Diets of European Neanderthals and Early Modern Humans." *Proceedings of the National Academy of Science of the United States of America* 106 (38): 16034–39.

Rimoli, C., C. N. Carducci, C. Dabas, C. Vescina, M. E. Quindimil, and A. Mascaró. 1991. "Relationship between Serum Concentrations of Flecainide and Fluoride in Humans." *Bolletine Chimico Farmaceutico* 130 (7): 279–82.

Ruan, Jianyan, and Ming H. Wong. 2001. "Accumulation of Fluoride and Aluminum Related to Different Varieties of Tea Plants." *Environmental Geochemistry and Health* 23 (1): 53–63.

Sala, Mike. 2013. "Stinkbug Salsa for the Iodine Deficient." *Chicago Reader*, October 14, 2013. http://www.chicagoreader.com/Bleader/archives/2013/10/14/stinkbug-salsa-for-the-iodine-deficient

Saunders, Milton. 1975. "Fluoride Toothpastes as a Cause of Acne-like Eruptions." *Archives of Dermatology* 111 (793): 1033–34. doi: 10.1001/archderm.1976.01630310079027.

Schaefer, Otto. 1971. "When the Eskimo Comes to Town." *Nutrition Today* 6:8–16. doi: 10.1097/00017285-197705000-00007.

Seamans, Frank. 1983. "Historical, Economic and Legal aspects of Fluoride." In *Fluorides: Effects on Vegetation, Animals, and Humans*. James Shupe, ed. Salt Lake City, Utah: Paragon Press.

Shea, J. J., S. M. Gillespie, and G. L. Waldbott. 1969. "Allergy to Fluoride." *Annals of Allergy*. 25: 388–391. As cited in "Allergy to Fluoride." Fluoride Action Network. April 17, 2012. http://fluoridealert.org/studies/shea-1967

Sigurdson, Tina. 2013. "Exposing the Cosmetics Cover-Up: True Horror Stories of Cosmetic Dangers." The Environmental Working Group. http://www.ewg.org/research/exposing-cosmetics-cover/true-horror-stories-of-cosmetic-dangers

Sigurdson, Tina, and Galen Roth. 2015. "Brazilian-Style Blowouts: Still Poisonous, Still in Salons." Environmental Working Group. http://www.ewg.org/enviroblog/2015/08/brazilian-style-blowouts-still-poisonous-still-salons

Simmons, Perez, and Howard D. Nelson. 1975. "Insects on Dried Fruits." Agriculture Handbook 464. U.S. Department of Agriculture, Agricultural Research Service. [Recreated and published as an Acrobat pdf in 2005, with an added list of updates and corrections, by Judy Johnson.] http://www.ars.usda.gov/is/np/insectsdriedfruits/insectsdriedfruits.pdf

"Skeletal Fluorosis in India and Its Relevance to the West." 2012. Fluoride Action Network. http://fluoridealert.org/articles/india-fluorosis

Smith, Robyn, Anna Braue, George A. Varigos, and Neil J. Mann. 2008a. "The Effect of a Low Glycemic Load Diet on Acne Vulgaris and the Fatty Acid

Composition of Skin Surface Triglycerides." *Journal of Dermatological Science* 50 (1): 41–52. doi: 10.1016/j.jdermsci.2007.11.005.

Smith, Robyn, Neil J. Mann, Anna Braue, Henna Mäkeläinen, and George A. Varigos. 2007a. "A Low-glycemic-load Diet Improves Symptoms in Acne Vulgaris Patients: A Randomized Controlled Trial." *American Journal of Clinical Nutrition* 86 (1): 107–15.

———. 2007b. "The Effect of a High-protein, Low Glycemic-load Diet Versus a Conventional, High Glycemic-load Diet on Biochemical Parameters Associated with Acne Vulgaris: A Randomized, Investigator-masked, Controlled Trial." *Journal of the American Academy of Dermatology* 57 (2): 247–56. doi: 10.1016/j.jaad.2007.01.046.

Smith, Robyn, Neil Mann, Henna Mäkeläinen, Jessica Roper, Anna Braue, and George Varigos. 2008b. "A Pilot Study to Determine the Short-term Effects of a Low Glycemic Load Diet on Hormonal Markers of Acne: A Nonrandomized, Parallel, Controlled Feeding Trial." *Molecular Nutrition and Food Research* 52 (6): 718–26. doi: 10.1002/mnfr.200700307.

"Sources of Fluoride: Pharmaceuticals." n.d. Fluoride Action Network. Accessed October 11, 2017, fluoridealert.org/issues/sources/pharmaceuticals/

Stanbury, John B., A. E. Ermans, P. Bourdoux, et al. 1998. "Iodine-Induced Hyperthyroidism: Occurrence and Epidemiology." *Thyroid* 8 (1): 83–100.

Stanley, Malcom M. 1949. "The Direct Estimation of the Rate of Thyroid Hormone Formation in Man. The Effect of the Iodide Ion on Thyroid Iodine Utilization." *Journal of Clinical Endocrinology* 9:941–54.

Stanley, Malcom M., and Edwin B. Astwood. 1949. "1-Methyl-2 -Mercaptoimidazole; An Antithyroid Compound Highly Active in Man." *Endocrinology* 44 (6): 588.

Stannard, J. G., Y. S. Shim, M. Kritsineli, P. Labropoulou, and A. Tsamtsouris. 1991. "Fluoride Levels and Fluoride Contamination of Fruit Juices." *Journal of Clinical Pediatric Dentistry* 16 (1): 38–40.

Statista. n.d. "Sales of the Leading Toothpaste Brands in the United States in 2014." Accessed September 10, 2015, https://www.statista.com/statistics /350439/us-supermarkets-toothpaste-dollar-sales

"Sulfuryl Fluoride: Pesticide Tolerance." Federal Register 70, no. 135 (2005): 40899–40908. Accessed February 17, 2017, http://www.epa.gov/fedrgstr /EPA-PEST/2005/July/Day-15/p13982.htm

Sulzberger, Marion B., and Sadie H. Zaidens. 1948. "Psychogenic Factors in Dermatological Disorders." *Medical Clinics of North America* 32 (3): 669–72.

Susheela, A. K., and Madhu Bhavnagar. 2002. "Reversal of Fluoride Induced Cell Injury through Elimination of Fluoride and Consumption of Diet Rich in Essential Nutrients and Antioxidants." *Developments in Molecular and Cellular Biochemistry* 37:335–40.

Thayer, Ann M. 2006. "Fabulous Fluorine." *Chemical and Engineering News* 84 (23): 15–24. http://pubs.acs.org/email/cen/html/060606071341.html

"The Story of Fluoridation." n.d. National Institute of Dental and Craniofacial Research. Accessed February 15, 2017, https://www.nidcr.nih.gov /OralHealth/Topics/Fluoride/TheStoryofFluoridation.htm

"The Universal Consensus on Sulfuryl Fluoride = Keep It Away from Food." 2013. Fluoride Action Network. http://fluoridealert.org/content/sf _consensus

Uhlenhake, Elizabeth, Brad Yentzer, and Steven Feldman. 2010. "Acne Vulgaris and Depression: A Retrospective Examination." *Journal of Cosmetic Dermatology* 9 (1): 59–63.

U.S. Department of Agriculture. 1972. "Air Pollutants Affecting the Performance of Domestic Animals." Agricultural Handbook No. 380. https://naldc.nal .usda.gov/naldc/download.xhtml?id=CAT72349227&content=PDF

———. 2005. "National Fluoride Database of Selected Beverages and Foods." Release 2. http://www.ars.usda.gov/SP2UserFiles/Place/80400525/Data /Fluoride/F02.pdf

———. n.d. "Petitioned Substances." Accessed October 8, 2017, http://www .ams.usda.gov/rules-regulations/organic/national-list/co

U.S. Public Health Service. 1974. "Fluoride: An Essential Mineral Nutrient." https://www.dentalwatch.org/usphs/ppb-67.pdf

Venturi, Sebastiano. 2011. "Evolutionary Significance of Iodine." *Current Chemical Biology* 5 (3): 155–62.

Vikoren, Torid, and Gudbrand Stuve. 1996. "Fluoride Exposure and Selected Characteristics of Eggs and Bones of the Herring Gull (Larus Argentatus) and the Common Gull (Larus Canus)." *Journal of Wildlife Diseases* 32 (2): 190–98.

Walters, Charles B., John C. Sherlock, William H. Evans, and John I. Read. 1982. "Dietary Intake of Fluoride in the United Kingdom and Fluoride Content of Some Foodstuffs." *Journal of the Science of Food and Agriculture* 34 (5): 523–28.

Warnakulasuriya, Saman, C. Harris, S. Gelbier, J. Keating, and T. Peters. 2002. "Fluoride Content of Alcoholic Beverages." *Clinica Chimica Acta* 320 (1–2): 1–4.

Warren, John, and Steven M. Levy. 2003. "Current and Future Role of Fluoride in Nutrition." *Dental Clinics of North America* 47:225–43. doi: 10.1016 /S0011-8532(02)00098-8

Wears, Adam. 2014. "Humpty Dumpty Was a Cannon Not an Egg." KnowledgeNuts. http://knowledgenuts.com/2014/01/08/humpty-dumpty -was-a-cannon-not-an-egg

Webster, Guy F. 2008. "Commentary: Diet and Acne." *Journal of the American Academy of Dermatology* 58 (5): 794–95.

Wedeen, R. P. 1989. "Were the Hatters of New Jersey 'Mad'?" *American Journal of Industrial Medicine* 16 (2): 225–33.

Weil, Andrew. 2005. "Worried About White Spots on Fingernails?" DrWeil. com. February 11, 2005. https://www.drweil.com/health-wellness /balanced-living/healthy-living/worried-about-white-spots-on-fingernails

Weinstein, Leonard. 1983. "Effects of Fluorides on Plants and Plant Communities: An Overview." In *Fluorides: Effects on Vegetation, Animals, and Humans.* James Shupe, ed. Salt Lake City, Utah: Paragon Press.

Weinstein, Leonard H., and A. Davison. 2004. *Fluorides in the Environment: Effects on Plants and Animals.* Cambridge, Mass: CABI Publishing.

White, Michael. 2009. *A Short Course in International Marketing Blunders: Mistakes Made by Companies that Should Have Known Better.* 3rd ed. Petaluma, CA: World Trade Press.

Whitford, Gary. 1990. "The Physiological and Toxicological Characteristics of Fluoride." *Journal of Dental Research* 69:539–49. doi: 10.1177/00220345900690S108.

Whitford, Gary, Richard S. Callan, and H.S. Wang. 1982. "Fluoride Absorption through the Hamster Cheek Pouch: a pH-Dependent Event." *Journal of Applied Toxicology* 2 (6): 303–6.

Whitford, Gary, F. C. Sampaio, P. Arneberg, and F. R. von der Fehr. 1999. "Fingernail Fluoride: A Method for Monitoring Fluoride Exposure." *Caries Research* 33 (6): 462–67.

Whyte, M. P., K. Essmyer, F. H. Gannon, and W. R. Reinus. 2005. "Skeletal Fluorosis and Instant Tea." *American Journal of Medicine* 118 (1): 78–82.

Wilson, Lawrence. 2011. *Sauna Therapy for Detoxification and Healing.* Prescott, Ariz: L.D. Wilson Consultants.

Wolff, Jan. 1969. "Iodide Goiter and the Parmacologic Effects of Excess Iodide." *American Journal of Medicine* 47 (1): 101–24.

Wolff, Jan, and Israel L. Chaikoff. 1948. "The Inhibitory Action of Iodide upon Organic Binding of Iodine by the Normal Thyroid Gland." *The Journal of Biological Chemistry* 172 (2): 855–56. http://www.jbc.org/content /172/2/855.full.pdf

Yeung, C. Albert, Lee Yee Chong, and Anne-Marie Glenny. 2015. "Fluoridated Milk for Preventing Tooth Decay." *Cochrane Database of Systematic Reviews*. September 3, 2015. http://www.cochrane.org/CD003876/ORAL _fluoridated-milk-preventing-tooth-decay

Zhou, L. Y., Z. D. Wei, and S. Z. Ldu. 1987. "Effect of Borax in Treatment of Skeletal Fluorosis." *Fluoride* 20 (1): 24–27.

Zipporah, Iheozor-Ejiofor Z., Helen V. Worthingon, Tanya Walsh, et al. 2015. "Water Fluoridation for the Prevention of Dental Caries." *Cochrane Database of Systematic Reviews* 6. doi: 10.1002/14651858.CD010856.pub2.

Index

Abraham, Guy, 174, 177, 181–83,
    189–93, 202
Accutane, 16–17
adolescent acne, 94, 176–77
adult acne, 13, 55–56, 60, 134, 163
Alcoa Corporation, 33–35, 37–38
alcohol, 27–28, 91. *See also* beer; wine
aluminum
    in cookware, 125
    in pesticides, 92
    in pollution, 25, 33, 35, 37, 42, 103
    in tea, 99
American Academy of Dermatology
    (AAD), 2, 59, 72
American Dental Association (ADA),
    40, 45, 51
amphibians, 220
Analysis of Competing Hypotheses
    (ACH), 179
anchovies, 107–8
anecdotal, 5, 7, 31, 53–57, 140,
    177
animal testing, 36, 73, 119, 183–84,
    193, 195
antifluoridation movement, 43,
    48–51, 77, 223–25, 228–29

antithyroid drugs, 188–91
apple cider vinegar, 19, 109, 149, 167
apricots, 119–20
Aquaria, 152–56
archaeology, 210–16, 218–19
arthritis, 74, 79, 81, 173. *See also*
    skeletal fluorosis
ASPCA's Animal Poison Control
    Center, 115–17
asthma, 12, 180, 182
Astwood, E. B., 187–88
Attention Deficit Hyperactivity
    Disorder (ADHD), 73
Australia, 14, 25, 27, 204, 212–13,
    216

bathing, 132–37, 160, 166
Battelle Laboratory, 119, 226
beauty products. *See* organic food and
    beauty products
beer, 28, 87, 90–91
bentonite clay, 167–68
benzoyl peroxide, 16–18, 71
Bernays, Edward, 42–45
bioaccumulation, 55–56, 75, 83,
    103–4, 106–7, 172–73

biomonitoring, 173
bone, 50, 55, 74–75, 104–8, 132,
    208. *See also* arthritis; skeletal
    fluorosis
borax, 195. *See also* boron
boron, 68–69, 195–96, 201
bottled water, 17, 22–23, 89, 133
brain damage, 17, 72–73, 121, 218,
    227. *See also* intelligence quotient;
    neurotoxicity of fluoride
branding. *See* marketing
Brita water filters, 90
Brockovich, Erin, 224–25
bromide, 67–68, 75, 121–22, 174,
    178, 187, 197–98
Brown, Halina, 134–36
Brownstein, David, 190, 196, 200
bureaucracy, 117–18, 128, 138, 146,
    176, 179, 182, 186, 224–25

California Department of Pesticide
    Regulation (CDPR), 92,
    113–15
Camellia sinensis. See tea
Canadian Dental Association, 50
canker sores, 60
cannibalism, 205
carcinogenicity, 145, 151, 227
caribou, 207–8
caries. *See cavities*
castor oil, 163
caveman regimen, 168
cavities
    and dental jargon, 40
    and fluoride, 32–36, 45, 47, 76,
        139, 198
    societies without, 205–6

celebrities
    with acne, 134, 160–62
    against fluoride, 225
Center for Disease Control (CDC)
    and chemicals used in fluoridation,
        24, 135
    on fluoride bioaccumulation, 57, 173
    guidelines on fluoride and drinking
        water, 22, 55, 88–89, 93, 105
    statements on fluoridation, 31, 225
cereal, 26, 28, 108–9, 111, 117
cetaceans, 219–20
chicken. *See* eggs; poultry products
chlorine, 67–68, 126, 181
chlorofluorocarbons, 126
chocolate, 10–11, 13, 30, 79
Cochrane Review Group, 36–37, 139,
    141
coconut oil, 19, 127, 149, 160, 164
Colquhoun, John, 49
comedones, 177–78
compressed air, 128–31
congressional hearings, 45, 226–27
Connett, Paul, 50–51
consumer confidence reports. *See*
    water quality reports
Cordain, Loren, 11–15, 25, 27–30, 61,
    81, 134
Crest toothpaste, 45–46. *See also*
    toothpaste
cretinism, 70, 182, 203, 206, 219
cryolite, 48, 70, 92–94, 106, 113–121
crystal ball technique. *See* thinking
    backwards exercise
cupping therapy, 165
cystic acne, 5, 17–18, 21–23, 53, 59,
    82–83, 158, 175, 197

dairy, 81, 94–98, 202, 205–7, 210.
    See also milk
DDT, 118, 224
Dean, H. Trendley, 33–34, 36,
    38–40, 42
dental fluorosis, 21, 33, 56–57
dental treatments. *See* fluoride dental
    treatments
depression, 58–67, 72, 74, 79, 81, 84,
    101, 170, 173
dermal absorption, 132–37
detoxification, 156–57, 166, 173,
    194–96, 198–201
dialysis, 132
Diaz, Cameron, 133–34
dogs, 36, 115–19, 220
Dow Chemical Company, 121–23
Dr. Strangelove, 31, 42
dulse, 199, 205. *See also* seaweed
DuPont, 35, 125–26

eggplant, 80, 115, 120
eggs, 103–4, 122, 182, 202, 208, 210,
    213, 221. *See also* fish eggs
Elf Atochem North America, 93,
    114
Environmental Protection Agency
    (EPA)
    and fluoridated drinking water, 30,
        49–50, 88–89, 93, 227
    and fluoride in air pollution, 24
    and fluoride pesticides, 105–6, 114,
        117–22
    and fluorinated chemicals used in
        manufacturing, 130
Environmental Working Group
    (EWG), 122, 131, 145–46

epiphany, 22–24, 52
Eskimos, 12, 29–31, 52, 204–5, 207,
    212–13
essential nutrients, 69–70, 182, 184,
    196
evolution, 215–17, 219–21
exfoliation, 164, 168

facial masks, 16, 161, 167, 169–70
Fallon, Sally, 178, 207
Farm Bill, 122–23
farming, 98, 113, 162
Farrow, Lynne, 180, 195–96
fast food, 134
Federal Food, Drug, and Cosmetic
    Act, 123, 145
fibromyalgia, 74, 190
Fiji, 205
filters, 89–90, 133
fingernails, 65–67, 81
Finland, 77–79
fish, 12, 28, 107–8, 111, 177, 209,
    211–13, 219. *See also* fish eggs;
    shellfish
fish eggs, 177, 194, 205, 207, 209–10
flame retardants, 75, 126, 131, 198
Flechas, Jorge, 175, 190, 217
fluoridation of the public water
    supply. *See also* antifluoridation
    movement
    chemicals used in, 22, 24–25, 56, 89
    as a conspiracy theory, 31, 42, 109
    in Europe, 36–37, 91
    history of, 29, 32, 34–46, 92
    naturally occurring, 88
    studies of, 34, 36–38, 72–73,
        76–79, 226–27

Fluoride Action Network (FAN), 51,
122, 218, 224

fluoride dental treatments, 21, 45–46,
57, 66, 82, 140–42

fluoride in the food supply, 26–31,
69–71, 87–100, 104–10, 114–15,
119–24

fluoride poisoning, 24, 67, 74, 79,
115–17, 121–22, 140–42

Fluorine Lawyers Committee, 37–38

FluoroCouncil, 126

fluorosis. *See* dental fluorosis; skeletal
fluorosis

fluorotechnology, 126, 130

Food and Drug Administration
(FDA), 89, 95, 97, 114–15, 117,
188

Fresno, 92–93, 100, 103, 111, 113,
115

fumigation, 121–23, 198

Ghent, Bill, 189–90

goiter, 70, 180–81, 183, 186–87, 203,
208–9

goitrogens, 185, 187, 189, 193, 198,
202. *See also* bromide; fluoride in
the food supply

Grand Rapids fluoridation trials, 34,
36, 38–39, 79

grapes, 91–93, 111–17, 120

Greek caveman talk, 56, 65, 148, 160

Guyenet, Stephan, 202

Hakala Research Laboratory, 197

half-life of fluoride, 172

halogens, 67–71, 193, 198, 201, 209

hatmaking, 101–2

heart palpitations, 195, 199

Heuer, Richards, 4, 176, 184, 203

hidradenitis suppurativa, 80

Hirzy, William, 50, 227–28

Homo floresiensis, 219

Homo neanderthalensis, 213, 218–19

Homo sapiens, 201–5, 211–24

hormones, 104, 144. *See also* thyroid
hormone

role in causing acne, 2, 13, 72, 81,
94, 97

Hurtado, Magdalena, 12–13, 15, 30

hydrofluorocarbon, 129

hydroponics, 100

hyperthyroidism, 71, 136, 183, 185,
187–88

hypoallergenic, 74, 163

hypothyroidism, 71–72, 189, 203, 219

hypotrichosis, 148

inflammation, 13–14, 25, 56

intelligence analysis, 3–4, 25, 53, 61,
75–76, 176–79, 184, 201–3, 222

intelligence quotient (IQ), 17, 73,
217–18

International Society for Fluoride
Research, 48

International Sugar Research
Foundation, 46–47

Internet, 65–67, 80, 119, 129, 131–32,
136, 140, 150, 161, 163, 173, 192,
226–27

Inuit, 11–12, 29–30, 207–8

iodine, 67–68, 70–73, 81, 226

history of, 179–92

role in evolutionary biology, 200–21

supplementation, 174–79, 192–200

iodine-loading test, 197–98
Iodine Project, 174–75, 178–79, 191, 193, 196–200
Iodoral, 199–200
isotretinoin. *See* Accutane

jojoba oil, 164
jubjub nuggets, 134
juice, 26, 90, 93–94

Kearns, Cristin, 46–47
kelp, 194, 205, 208–9, 212–13. *See also* seaweed
Kelp Highway Hypothesis, 212–13
Kennerly, William, 141
Kettering Laboratory of Applied Physiology, University of Cincinnati, 35–36, 38
kidneys, 74, 115, 132, 186, 208
Kitavan Islanders, 12–13, 28–30, 52, 79, 87
Kocher, Theodore, 182–83
Kryocide, 92–93. *See also* cryolite

Langley, Samuel, 1, 5–7
language, 3, 213, 217–18
leukonychia, 65–66
levothyroxine, 189
Limeback, Hardy, 50, 57
Lindeberg, Staffan, 12–13, 15, 30
Lugol's solution, 181, 183, 199
lymphatic system, 20, 36, 155–58, 160, 165–66, 170–71
lymph drainage therapy, 20, 158

Madrid Statement, 126
magnesium, 107, 196

Mann, Neil, 27, 29
Marcus, William, 49–50, 227
Marean, Curtis, 214–16
marketing, 38–46, 111–12, 146, 148
Masai, 206–7
massage. *See* lymph drainage therapy
matcha tea, 100
McCaughey, Peyton, 121
McCay, Frederick, 33–34
McConaughey, Matthew 160–62, 164
mechanically deboned meat (MDM), 104–6
melasma, 18, 71
Mellon Institute of Industrial Research, University of Pittsburgh, 35
mercurial poisoning, 73, 101–2, 224
methyl bromide, 121–22
milk, 11, 26, 28, 70, 94–98, 182, 206–8, 221. *See also* dairy
milk fluoridation, 139
mink oil, 160–62, 164, 179
moisturizer, 16, 19, 145, 149–50
Mommypotamus, 160, 163, 169
monocropping, 113, 115–16
Monte Verde, 210–11
Mullenix, Phyllis, 49, 72–73

National Caries Program, 47
National Institute of Dental and Craniofacial Research (NIDCR), 32–34, 37, 39, 42, 46, 57
National Institute of Dental Research (NIDR), 34, 39, 47
National Institute of Health (NIH), 33, 186–87, 218

National Organic Standards, 93–94
National Raisin Reserve, 112–13
National Research Council (NRC), 107, 172
National Toxicology Program (NTP), 227
neurotoxicity of fluoride, 49, 72–73, 202, 218, 227
nightshades, 80–81
nonstick pans. See Teflon

oats, 26, 108–9, 205
oil cleansing, 160–65, 170
organic food and beauty products, 93–94, 100, 106–7, 109, 120, 123–24, 148, 164
osteomalacia, 132
ovaries, 71, 186, 190
Oz, Mehmet, 153–56, 225

paleo diet, 14, 25, 28, 79, 134, 178, 202–3, 205, 219
perioral dermatitis, 56, 82
Peru, 139, 187, 207–9, 212–13
pesticides, 27, 70, 83, 107, 109–10, 115–17. See also cryolite; methyl bromide; sulfuryl fluoride
petition to end fluoridation, 228–29
pharmaceuticals, 2, 72, 170, 202. See also Accutane
  with fluoride, 24, 124–25
  for the thyroid, 187–92
phosphate fertilizer industry, 24–25, 70, 225. See also pollution from airborne fluorides
pineal gland, 71–72, 106, 173
Pinnacle Point, 214–16

Polk County, 24
pollution from airborne fluorides, 24, 34–35, 37–38, 42, 48, 50, 70, 225. See also aluminum in pollution
popcorn, 126–27
potatoes, 27–28, 80, 109, 112
poultry products, 82–83, 104–7, 172
prenatal, 73
Price, Weston A., 178, 204–10, 213
Proactiv, 16–17
ProFume, 121, 123
Prozac, 124
prunes, 113, 196
PubMed, 106

qigong, 158
quinoa, 109–10

raisins, 28, 110–24, 179, 196
randomized controlled trials, 7, 14, 27
reciprocity, 27
restaurants, 86, 104, 108, 120
reverse osmosis, 22, 90. See also filters
rheumatoid arthritis, 74. See also arthritis; skeletal fluorosis
rice, 12, 26, 28, 108–9
Roholm, Kaj, 48

salicylic acid, 16
salt
  fluoridated, 138–39
  iodized, 181, 185
  sea salt, 107, 127, 196
saltwater, 107, 137, 141, 153, 155–56
San Joaquin Valley, 92–93, 110, 113–14, 120

sardines, 107

saunas, 166, 169

Schaefer, Otto, 11–12, 29–30

Scotchgard, 125, 127, 131

seafood, 107–8, 176, 182, 204–5, 207–8, 213–15. *See also* fish; seaweed; shellfish

seaweed, 174–75, 177, 180, 187, 190, 194, 198, 205–7, 209–10, 215. *See also* dulse; kelp

sebum, 2, 167

selenium, 68, 196–97, 199

shellfish, 107, 177, 205, 212–15, 219

Shirli and Larry, 129, 131, 134

skeletal fluorosis, 30, 55, 79, 99, 195–96, 198

Skin Deep Database, 146

Society for Investigative Dermatology, 10–11, 13

sodium lauryl sulfate (SLS), 133

soft drinks, 13–14, 27–28, 30, 90

status quo, 44, 118, 128

steam machine, 165–66

stinkbugs, 208

strigils, 160, 164, 168

sugar, 13–14, 25, 30, 46–47, 81, 204

suicide, 59–61

sulfuryl fluoride, 105, 121–23

Switzerland, 138–39, 182–83, 185, 206

Synthroid, 189

tea, 30–31, 70, 90, 99–101, 103, 198

Teflon, 125–26, 131, 144

testosterone, 13

thinking backwards exercise, 202–5, 221

thyroid gland, 70–71, 136, 175, 178, 180–89, 192, 199, 202, 208. *See also* hyperthyroidism; hypothyroidism

thyroid hormone, 71–72, 184, 207, 220

tobacco, 30, 43–44, 224

toothpaste, 18, 22, 24, 41, 45–46, 79, 82, 122, 132, 188

Toxic Substances Control Act (TSCA), 127, 130

TumTum trees, 138

turkey. *See* poultry products

ungulates, 219

USDA National Fluoride Database of Selected Beverages and Foods, 91, 96, 97, 110

U.S. Public Health Service (PHS), 38, 69, 76, 82, 102, 226

U.S. Senate Subcommittee on Wildlife, Fisheries, and Drinking Water, 228

Vienna Convention, 121

Vikane, 121, 123

Vodder, Emil and Estrid, 158

Waldbott, George, 22, 48–49, 76

water quality reports, 25, 88–89

Webster, Guy *"Sassypants,"* 94

Weil, Andrew, 65–66

well water, 57, 88

Western Grapeleaf Skeletonizers, 91–92, 110, 113

Whistleblower Protection Act, 49, 227

Wikipedia, 54, 66, 95, 104, 167, 183

wine, 28, 87, 91–93, 100, 105,
110–11, 114–15
Wolff–Chaikoff effect, 183–91, 193
World Health Organization (WHO),
36, 139, 203, 217
World War I, 111, 181

World War II, 24, 37, 98, 102,
111
Wright brothers, 1, 6–7, 193, 224

yerba maté, 30, 100
yoga, 19, 158, 200

BOOKS OF RELATED INTEREST

Colloidal Silver
The Natural Antibiotic
by Werner Kühni and Walter von Holst

Shungite
Protection, Healing, and Detoxification
by Regina Martino

The Book of Tapping
Emotional Acupressure with EFT
by Sophie Merle

The Acid-Alkaline Diet for Optimum Health
Restore Your Health by Creating pH Balance in Your Diet
by Christopher Vasey, N.D.

Total Life Cleanse
A 28-Day Program to Detoxify and Nourish the Body, Mind, and Soul
by Jonathan Glass, M.Ac., C.A.T.

Black Cumin
The Magical Egyptian Herb for Allergies, Asthma, and Immune Disorders
by Peter Schleicher, M.D. and Mohamed Saleh, M.D.

Ayurveda: A Life of Balance
The Complete Guide to Ayurvedic Nutrition and Body Types with Recipes
by Maya Tiwari

The Miracle of Regenerative Medicine
How to Naturally Reverse the Aging Process
by Elisa Lottor, Ph.D., H.M.D.
Foreword by Judi Goldstone, M.D.

INNER TRADITIONS • BEAR & COMPANY
P.O. Box 388
Rochester, VT 05767
1-800-246-8648
www.InnerTraditions.com

Or contact your local bookseller